Cancer:

HOW TO MAKE SURVIVAL WORTH LIVING

Coping With Long Term Effects of Cancer Treatment

By: Ms Patricia R Wheeler M.A.

D1533778

Cover image from the original painting "Heron Greets the Day" by Madeline McMurray, Eureka, California.

For my mother, Isabelle Anderson Dolan,
Who gave me her time;

For my friend, Leslie Bowman Marcus,
Who knew all about short time;

And for Christina Pirruccello Rosales,
Who was taken long before her time.

Acknowledgments

This book would never have been written without the support and encouragement of Michael Pirruccello, M.D. As busy as he is, he took time to read and comment on every chapter as I delivered them to him. He has now taken the position of Executive Director of our medical center's extended hours operation, and I know all his patients miss him as much as I do. Dr. Alali, Dr. Chew, Dr. Erba, and Dr. Koch, as well as my dentist, Dr. Amy Tran, and Dr. Terry Lee, my chiropractor, will never know how much I appreciate them. I am so grateful for the encouragement of my sister, Madeline McMurray, and the patience of her husband, David McMurray, who stood by as we worked through my ideas and her feedback. Madeline also has my never-ending gratitude for use of the painting, "Heron Greets the Day". I fell in love with it the moment I saw it in her studio, and I am thrilled to have it on the cover of this book. Thanks, too, to my dear friend, advisor and "pixel expert", William Marcus, without whose efforts we wouldn't have either the heron or the brain. Gratitude goes always to my darling Kimmie for everything she is and does, and to her and Allison for helping me through my treatments. I couldn't have done any of that without the aid and comfort of my sister, the Reverend Celia Scott, who ministered to me and also taught my classes when I wasn't able. Thanks as well to all my students who have been through this journey with me; you guys are awesome. Finally, great thanks to my medical, dental, and CreateSpace teams and to all those, known and unknown, who helped me on the path to wellness, print, and transformation from the feisty little hummingbird to the resilient heron who confidently greets every new day.

Table of Contents

Preface

When I stepped out of the shower, I happened to turn at just the right angle that allowed me to see the mass in my breast. I remember thinking, "So that's what's wrong with me." I had known for several weeks that I was sick with something very serious, and how people scoffed when I said I thought I had cancer. Now, I had at least tentative proof, but that wasn't a good thing to be right about!

I gave myself a day to get used to the idea that there were going to be some big changes in my life, and then I called my doctor. He wasn't available that morning, so I saw his P.A., and the minute she palpated the mass, she was off down the hall, and in seconds, Dr. Pirruccello was by my side. After a quick examination—remember, we could see this "lump"—he said, "We're going to treat this like it's an aggressive cancer until we find out that it isn't." And I nodded, because I trusted him.

The next day I saw the radiologist who thought it might just be a cyst that had filled with fluid. I've had fibrocystic breasts since I was in my 20's, and I'd had my annual mammogram just five months earlier, so it wasn't an unreasonable thought. He asked the nurse to bring him a biopsy tray, which contained an enormous needle with which he began to extract fluid that was, indeed, contained in the cyst. He drained it three times and expressed some frustration that it was still hard. That meant we had to go to the next step, which was a biopsy. That hurt like the dickens. It turned out the tumor was behind the cyst, so as the cyst was drained, the doctor was then dealing with the mass itself.

The next day my mother and I returned to the radiologist's office to get the report. He said "The news is not good. Do you have a preference in surgeons?" I told him I wanted Dr. Dominic Erba, whom I knew to be a good and honest surgeon from his having operated on my mother for a carotid artery blockage. Then we headed for my mother's porch where we sat and watched hummingbirds protecting their territory the whole rest of that day. There was absolutely no better thing I could have done.

Hummingbirds are pretty special. As tiny as they are they defend their territory from a couple of neighbors away by puffing themselves up to look like really big birds. Then if another hummer dares to head for their flowers and feeders, they swoop down, little wings churning, and chase the invader away. I liked the image and used it often as I went through my treatment.

I had invasive, Stage III breast cancer. A mastectomy was the only option for me, and I chose not to have reconstruction because I just couldn't go through anything that wasn't necessary. By then I'd had enough surgeries in my life, and today's mastectomy is nothing like the original. I have one straight line scar across the side of my chest that extends into my armpit. That's all. I wear a prosthesis, and I don't know that anyone who didn't know about my choice could ever tell.

The tumor was stage III, 8.5 centimeters, and I had cancer in 19 of the 27 lymph nodes Dr. Erba could reach. It was, indeed, an aggressive cancer, so it would be chemotherapy and radiation for me. Dr. Erba's original opinion, even with a tumor that big and that many "dirty" nodes, was that the cancer was systemic, but not metastasized. I chose to believe him because he's the one who had seen the things, and he had seen who knows how many of both things in his surgical career. And I trusted him. The first CT scan, six weeks later proved him right.

After the surgery, the healing, and the scan, I was off to the UC Davis Cancer Center for chemotherapy and radiation. There I met Dr. Helen Chew, one of the best women and doctors I know. The people at the Med Center (like my doctors at home) are my kind of people, because they tell the truth about what you can expect, what they know, and what they don't know. The clinical nurses and the staff in the infusion center are honest and kind and often funny. The students who are doing oncology rounds are a little tentative and very respectful, and I can't help but love them for what they are doing.

About a year after I finished with radiation (two years after my first diagnosis), my team released me to work as hard as I wanted and could to lose the weight I'd gained during treatment, and I got busy. I ate well and exercised a lot and spent hours doing pretty heavy work in my garden. And I began to lose weight—but not from my belly. One day, after my exercise routine, I raised my shirt and said to my mother, "Look at this", and she said, "You look pregnant". Well, that wasn't likely, so I knew we had a problem once again.

I called Dr. Pirruccello's office, and he had me come right in, immediately sent me over for a sonogram, and told me to come back that afternoon. Which I did. He came into the room and said, "It's on the ovary, and it's big". So I fired up my little hummingbird wings and flew over to Dr. Koch, the gynecologist, who agreed that it was there and it was big, and a CA-125 was ordered up. Well, the CA-125 is an important test for ovarian cancer, but it isn't yet very reliable. Mine never got above level three, so we had no reason to think that cancer was involved this time. But it was. I laugh about the good Dr. Koch coming in post-surgery and saying, "We found a little bit of cancer on the surface of that tumor", and my replying, "So, we'll just do a little bit of chemo, okay?". And he said, "No. We'll do six rounds, and I'm making an appointment for you to see our new oncologist". I just pulled the covers over my sparsely haired head and groaned.

And that's how I met Dr. Alborz Alali, another fine physician, kind and good humored and honest. There would be no radiation this time, but the chemo was harder for me to handle. I had white cell drops, delays, I couldn't work all the time, and I felt just plain lousy. Between the third and fourth sessions, I told Dr. Alali I just couldn't do it anymore. I just put my head down on his desk and said I had to stop. What a guy! He just kept saying in his way, "You can do this; you're almost done; you won't quit now….." until I finally raised my head, and agreed. And the hummingbird and I flew some more, a little slower this time, but still defending our territory against this damned invader.

I'm ten years away from that first experience, and eight years away from big (soccer ball sized) ovarian tumor with early stage cancer. I say with an eight plus centimeter breast mass and a soccer ball on my ovary. no one can accuse me of not making big tumors—but there's no award for that! And I hope I never get another chance to beat my records! I am a survivor because right now, and for some time, I've been cancer free. But I still fight every day to manage what the Mayo Clinic calls the "late effects of cancer treatment". And you will need to do that, too. So, be like the hummingbird: puff yourself up, churn those wings, and get ready to chase away every single side or after or late or long-term effect of cancer treatment that tries to take over your territory! The quality of your life, the contents of your wallet, and your sense of overall well-being depend on it.

Patricia R. Wheeler, M.A.

Introduction

I was 61 years old the first time I came down with cancer just before the terrorist acts on the World Trade Center in 2001. I have been absolutely unwilling to accept the idea that the things that happened to me since September 17 of that year, the day of my first surgery, and continue to this day are a result of my growing older. I certainly believed that if I were inclined to hypochondria, the ongoing complaints I have would have developed with any one of the earlier five or six major surgeries I've undergone in my life. I believed people who survive cancer treatment remain forever thereafter cancer patients. I believed there are long term after effects to cancer treatment, and I kept asking questions and searching for answers because I wouldn't settle for "you're not getting any younger" and "we all have problems as we age"!

We're all pretty comfortable talking about the side effects of chemotherapy and radiation treatments for cancer. We don't talk much at all about the after, late or long-term effects. My chemo brain was understandable for others when I was in therapy, but once the infusion port was removed, my ability to remember names should have returned. And when it didn't, it was because I was older. Did that mean I was supposed to accept approaching senility? If I had the ability to remember names before chemo, and I lost it while I was in chemo, and it didn't return after chemo, then how can anyone simply deduce that my chemo related memory loss was gone and my ongoing memory loss was suddenly related to advancing years?

Sometimes if we complain about the after effects, relating them to our cancer treatment, we create anxiety for ourselves because, as Bernie Siegal has written, our "spouse, friends and relatives unite in the conviction that it's time for you to get on with your life. [You are a survivor], and they want you to act normally because they believe you should have learned to live with your symptoms by now". It all boils down, it seems to me, to COUNT YOUR BLESSINGS! YOU'RE ALIVE!

But now I have found what I needed to be able to write this book! According to the Mayo Clinic, "Late effects are side effects of cancer treatment that become apparent after your treatment has ended. Cancer survivors might experience late effects of cancer treatment a few months after treatment is completed or years later… [S]ide effects that start during your cancer treatment and linger for months or years after are called long-term side effects".

You can't imagine how relieved I was to finally find an authoritative article that supported my certainty that the symptoms I have are related to my cancer treatment and not to my age! I was in one condition when I went into treatment for my first cancer, and I was different when my treatment ended. I was even more different after treatment for my second cancer. I am a survivor, but for me that means I had cancer, and now I live with the on-going effects of the treatment of that disease. The Mayo Clinic staff writes: "You might be surprised to know that side effects can continue after your cancer treatment or even develop several years later." One of those things that was recently announced is a clear connection between chemotherapy and diabetes.

And so, I'm writing this "Alphabet Soup" of my own experience in an effort to provide you, your friends, family and associates, as well as your medical teams and the other patients they serve with answers to your questions about some of the late effects of cancer treatment and some of the things you can do about them. I hope it helps.

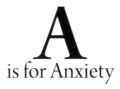

A
is for Anxiety

A nxiety is, according to the Columbia University on-line encyclopedia, anticipatory tension or vague dread persisting in the absence of a specific threat; in contrast to fear, which is a realistic reaction to actual danger, anxiety is generally related to an unconscious threat   Anxiety may well be the most overwhelming problem post treatment cancer patients endure. The operating theaters and their surgeries, the infusion centers with their hanging bags of chemotherapy and platelets, the radiation departments with their rotating tables and robotic arms, and even the rows of pill bottles lined up on our tables have engendered anxiety in us during our treatment. After treatment, the absence of the support team alone may cause anxiety to rise. We are glad to be out of it, and at the same time, we are afraid to go it alone.

Cancer patients begin every phase and aspect of their treatment protocol with anxiety because it's all unknown. The anxiety eases as each step is carefully explained and we have the opportunity to ask questions. The anxiety is complete when we have accomplished the test and feel relief at having done it and even having a story to tell. "That wasn't so bad", we say. Or "That was just awful; I hated it; I hope I never have to go through that again". Either way, the knowing relieves the anxiety, and we find ourselves back in a time of peace if not exactly total comfort. And if we do have to do it again, we know we can handle it, and our confidence and self-esteem rise again.

We do that all the way through the therapy process—through diagnosis, through surgery, through chemotherapy, through radiation, and during follow-up care. With every step we grow anxious, and with every step, we get through and experience a kind of relief. Then as each step is done once, we feel much less anxious when we have to do it again.

According to the American Cancer Society, however, "…people can feel distress at any time after cancer diagnosis and treatment, even many years after the cancer is treated. As their health situations change, people with cancer must cope with new stressors along with the old". So, imagine you're three years out of treatment and doing very well. You are a survivor! You probably still get a little anxious if you're having semi-annual scans and blood tests, but unless there's no reason to suspect a recurrence, you can handle it.

But anxiety still arises when we don't know what's going on, and from the moment you suspected you had cancer, there's been a lot of unknown stuff going on. When we don't know what to expect, then anxiety sets in. Fear is normal. Fear is sane. A character in a book I read recently said, "Being scared kept me awake. Kept me on my toes. Kept me alive." And that's true of us who have survived cancer treatment. We have to be on our toes to be truly alive; we have to be awake to know what's going on with us! The cancer is over; now it's up to us.

So, with that in mind, imagine that you're humming along in full survivor mode, and you wake up one morning with an almost unbearable pain in your hip. Suddenly you are overwhelmed again by anxiety because you don't know what's going on . The questions and doubts begin again, but these are new ones. "What caused that?" "What did I do to myself to cause that?" "Has the cancer spread?" "Maybe I wasn't really clear of it after all." And with your anxiety you take some aspirin or ibuprofen and try to put the pain out of your mind. You do a little exercise to try to "work it out". You stretch and you move and you meditate, and most of all, you say nothing to anyone about it. You're certainly not going to bother your oncologist with it; he/she is too busy with sick people to worry about a survivor. You're not going to pester your primary care doc with every little twinge that comes along—you're cancer free, and this is nothing. You surely aren't going to mention it to anyone in your family who are just getting over the frights of your treatment, because after all, what is there to tell? Your hip hurts. It's as simple as that; nothing more to it.

If you are body-minded, you might tell yourself that if it keeps up, then maybe you'll call your masseuse or your chiropractor and get a massage or an adjustment. "That'll do it" you tell yourself. We'll just wait and see. Then, lo and behold! It all changes. The next day the pain is gone. "See", you say to yourself, "it was nothing". The relief you feel this time is over the fact that you didn't make a fool of yourself by complaining to anyone about that little twinge you had in your hip.

You stay relaxed over the next few days, occasionally shaking your head at how you got yourself all afraid and anxious about nothing more than a little ache in your hip. Then a few days later, you're awakened from sleep by that same sharp pain you had before! It's so bad this time it would cause you to sit straight up in bed if only you could move. And if your partner wakes too, you say, "It's nothing. dear. Go back to sleep". When you can, you get up to take some aspirin or ibuprofen, and you hope that will take care of it—"It did before" you tell yourself. You walk a bit, working it out; you stretch, you breathe, and all the while you're fighting that one anxious thought: "Has it come back?"

The cancer probably hasn't come back, but the pain very likely is related to your cancer and your treatment. Many cancer patients who have been out of treatment for some length of time, may want to "put on a happy face", not merely for the benefit of others, but because of the anxiety itself! They may try to hide the anxiety because to admit it might mean that their most basic fear, a recurrence of their cancer, needs to be hidden not only from those around them, but from themselves as well.

As the pain in your hip becomes more severe, though, you will very likely get to the point of these lines from Byron Shelley's poem "Stanzas Written in Despair" before you make an appointment with your doctor or reach the date of your regularly scheduled follow-up because you are afraid they won't believe you or you'll be deemed a hypochondriac:

> *Alas! I have no hope nor health,*
> *Nor peace within nor calm around…*

That feeling of despair will ultimately give you the courage to speak up, and after you get through the questions about how often the pain occurs, how long the pain lasts, whether you have pain at that moment, and when you do have pain, where does it stand on a 1 to 10 numerical scale, chances are you'll be asked what you did to yourself to cause it.

Or someone will, not unkindly, suggest that you're not as young as you used to be, and conclude your pain is related to aging, certainly not to the cancer or its treatment that you had years before. You might be given a stronger ibuprofen prescription, and applications of heat and ice (either or both) might be recommended. They might order up a bone density test which, if you aren't yet in your 70's and you are reasonably well nourished, will probably show you have pre-osteoporosis. They might give you medication for osteoporosis which can have negative side effects such as making the bones rigid and thus fragile in a way quite different from a lack of density.

So you go away from your appointment feeling a little ashamed for not living up to your courageous reputation as a survivor. You make a vow to ignore that anxiety, get into the gym, build yourself up, and not whine anymore. You've reached the point where you say to yourself something like the words of the great Dylan Thomas: "Someone's boring me. I think it's me." Then when you try whatever you try and the pain persists, you just accept it as a condition of getting older and do the best you can to talk yourself out

3

of worrying, not realizing that anxiety can develop years after you're out of cancer treatment for no apparent reason at all.

But your acceptance of the notion that your pain and the accompanying anxiety is really nothing at all will, of course, make it all into a self-fulfilling prophecy, for if you aren't able to find permanent relief from that hip pain, you soon will begin to give into it. It will be an ever-present aspect of your consciousness. You will begin to favor that leg, even as you pray for the pain to go away. Your posture will change. Your walk will be different. You'll begin to limit your activities. You won't dance anymore, or bend over so much, and certainly not lift heavy objects, and before long, you will be moving as though you were, indeed, old. If you feel old, you will begin to look old, and everyone around you will agree that the cancer certainly took a lot out of you.

That sad scenario will lead to further problems that are not related to your cancer. Your confidence will be affected. You'll begin to worry about your looks. You'll adjust to a more "age-appropriate" style. You'll wonder if your still young, robust husband will find his way to a younger woman. You'll slow down on your job, no matter what it is. The fact is, you are in pain and you are growing older. You cannot deny that. And facing your natural mortality will be quite different from the ways you dealt with the idea of cancer caused mortality.

While you may in time handle your hip pain, other things may well arise that take you into anxiety, which is a complex condition that can "bleed" into rage, depression or trauma, so it can be very serious, especially if it becomes chronic. Anxiety is more than a bad mood. It is a complex condition that requires medical attention, and I can't stress enough that it can develop even years out of cancer treatment.

Another potential long lasting effect of chemotherapy identified by the Mayo Clinic, Northwestern University Feingold School of Medicine and others, is pain, and not just pain in the hip. These episodes of pain can occur day or night, regularly or sporadically, whether you've worked too hard or not hard enough, whether you've walked, or lifted, or carried or sat in a chair or stretched out on the floor. Sometimes the pain is severe; sometimes it's tolerable. And when a long term survivor of cancer feels unexplained pain, anxiety will surely follow.

Because anxiety is usually considered to be situational and temporary or of long standing, as in the case of generalized anxiety disorder, the usual response is to refer the patient to a professional in the field of psychology. That person, quite frequently, will lean toward medication to help the patient. Proper medication is an extremely effective tool. But in the case of cancer treatment after effects, the physicians involved all need to understand that these manifestations of the symptoms of anxiety most likely are solidly connected to that treatment and not something out of a Freudian diagnostic tool. They also need to know that medications must be closely monitored in long term cancer survivors, because they may affect us in ways different from the expected norm. Some of the new psychotropic medications can be very effective; others can be more debilitating than the anxiety itself because if you already have long term chemo brain, you certainly do not want to complicate matters with medication that has the potential to degrade your cognitive abilities, which may already be affected.

When they made all those suggestions in the hope of helping you with your anxiety and your pain, your doctors meant no harm. Information on anxiety and pain in long term survivors is not yet commonly found in oncology journals, so your physicians may well not be aware yet of how anxiety can arise in cancer patients even years after they have completed treatment. So it's up to you to stay actively involved in all the processes so that you take control of your own psychosocial treatment. Nothing is more important.

By the way, that hip pain you had was probably indeed related to your cancer treatment. It's a common problem for long term survivors, and it can usually be managed nicely with a dietary supplement of 1500 milligrams of calcium and 600 milligrams of Vitamin D every day. That's all it takes.

When I learned that, my anxiety quickly turned to irritation. I was not as patient and understanding of the physicians' problems with a lack of knowledge then, and I found myself quoting the words of Maxine Waters in Brian Lanker's beautiful book of photography entitled, "I Dream a World". Waters said, "I have a right to my anger, and I don't want anybody telling me I shouldn't be, that it's not nice to be, and that something's wrong with me because I get angry." If that's where you find yourself, you can turn that anger into positive energy and use it to make a difference. The sky, Chicken Little, isn't falling after all.

It takes more than understanding Chicken Little's mistake, though, to manage anxiety and pain. Although the sky probably isn't falling, you do need some more particular information about anxiety and pain and other long lasting effects of cancer treatment, because your doctor is going to need your help in understanding the concept. You can become a leader in helping others understand what long term cancer survivors need in terms of continued care.

Be like Henny Penney and ask every question you can think of, and provide information that you have learned from this book and other sources so you can begin to create a conversation, and with that you can be sure that no one will be likely to prove Chicken Little to be right.

B
is for Body

I can't say that my body has ever cooperated with me. When Marilyn Monroe represented the feminine ideal, I looked like Twiggy. Then when Twiggy, who really was built like a stick, became popular, I was on my way to a more Monroe-like model. By my mid-30s, though, I was just about right in my eyes. And then when I was 60, I lost my breast to cancer.

I sometimes feel sad over the loss of my Monroe-oriented body. I remember once, at the beginning of the breast cancer awareness movement, seeing a picture of a whole group of single breasted women of all ages, races and sizes, proudly (it seemed) baring their chests for the camera. I remember being moved by the drama of their losses, but I felt so sad for them.

I miss the body that used to work me, walk me and dance me. I miss the way my body moved me through the world with hardly a care. Now in many ways, my body is a separate sort of self—one that I must constantly monitor and watch out for. (It's a lot like having a little kid to take care of!) I think I won't ever get used to it. At the same time, like with a little kid, I'm not willing to give in to its demands either! But I have had to learn to feed my body, dress my body, move my body, and generally treat my body in a whole new set of different ways. So I had to find a new celebrity image to relate to, one that would fit my philosophy professor self and this new body of mine. So I'm working on a Katherine Hepburn look, which fits my turtleneck and jeans wardrobe and my slower more cautious progress through the world. I have to lose a bit more belly fat to make the model work, and I'm sure the very sophisticated Ms. Hepburn would have been horrified by the jeans, but it's what I'm going for anyway.

So body image is important to me and I think it must be important to you, as well. And because of that, while this is a book about the long term after effects of cancer *treatment*, especially chemotherapy and radiation, I don't think I can do a chapter on the body without talking a little bit about breast reconstruction right out of the gate. So here goes.

Whether or not to have breast reconstruction after a mastectomy—or even a lumpectomy these days—is something that needs to be discussed by every woman with her medical team before her cancer surgery. The two types of procedure, flap and implant, are quite different and have different results. The flap procedure involves molding a new breast using tissue from another part of your body—back, buttocks or stomach. When that skin and body fat are removed, the shape of the "donor" location is changed, less so in the case of the stomach than the others. (Some plastic surgeons even suggest that with that procedure you get two for the price of one: a new breast and a tummy tuck!) The implant procedure involves inserting a saline or silicone implant into a space between the skin and the chest wall. The new procedures for "repairing" the defect caused by a lumpectomy, followed by radiation, involves transferring fat and tissue from donor sites.

The flap procedure, using the stomach as the donor site, called a TRAM flap procedure, is becoming the most popular, although it can, as the American Cancer Society reports "…reduce belly strength, and may not be possible in women who have had abdominal tissue removed in previous surgeries".

But all of the ins and outs of the various procedures and what's necessary to make the decision, are not for me to discuss here. I encourage anyone who is considering breast reconstruction to read the American Cancer Society's paper, "Breast Reconstruction After Mastectomy". It is a treasure of information!

Despite my sadness about the loss of my breast, I chose not to have reconstruction, and would not have it now, although it is almost always available to mastectomy patients even years out of treatment. Reconstruction has its own appearance problems and could never replicate what I looked like before, so I would still have been sad over the loss of my former body. And there were serious medical reasons not to have reconstruction at the time of my mastectomy.

I had aggressive Stage IIIB breast cancer which we knew from the outset, because of my rapidly growing fist-sized tumor, would require both chemotherapy and radiation. Radiation can have dramatic effects on the skin, and radiation can interfere with a successful reconstruction. Because of that, most physicians recommend that reconstruction in cases like mine begin a year after completion of radiotherapy to allow for complete healing.

If immediate reconstruction is the goal, the insertion of expanders begins immediately after the cancer surgery. Then the reconstruction, whichever plan is adopted, requires several procedures up to and including reconstruction of the nipple/areola complex, which is optional. There can be long term complications with breast reconstruction, including hardening of an implant or a shifting of the tissue from a flap procedure. Each of these long term complications requires more surgery if they develop. I simply could not bear the idea of any more surgeries.

And, as it turned out, I had to have a second surgery to correct bleeding problems the day after my mastectomy. If skin expanders had been in place, that would have been a complication already. Then two years later I had to have another surgery for my ovarian cancer, and that would have been right about the time all the procedures involved in reconstruction would have begun because of the recommendations on healing after radiation. I was confident that by the time two years passed—one of treatment and one of healing—I would be accustomed to having only one breast and wearing a prosthesis. (These days you can even have a prosthesis custom made to match your remaining breast--I might look into that!)

I never worried about a loss of sexual intimacy as a consequence of the loss of my breast, not because I wasn't involved in a romantic relationship at the time, but because I always felt--and still feel--that anyone who couldn't work through all of this with me wasn't the sort of partner I wanted in my life! But I understand that not all women agree with me, so I recommend these articles from the Breastcancer.org website: "Accepting the Nude You", dated October 19, 2010; "Single Women: Finding Your Way", dated July 28, 2008 and "Beyond Intercourse", dated July 9, 2011.

Through all of this, and all the other things I want to talk with you about, one thing becomes clear: the French writer, Marcel Proust, was absolutely right when he wrote "It is in moments of illness that we are compelled to recognize that we live not alone but chained to a creature of a different kingdom, whole worlds apart, who has no knowledge of us and by whom it is impossible to make ourselves understood: our body."

And as it turns out, it is not only in "moments of illness" that cancer treatment survivors are pushed around by our bodies. The long-term effects of chemotherapy and radiation affect the body long after cancer treatment is completed. Some of them involve pain, fatigue, nausea, stiffness, balance, dryness of skin, eyes, and mucosal tissue, cataracts, neuropathy of hands and feet, numbness, muscle cramping, phantom pains and many others. I'm going to save some of those for other more specific chapters, but I do want to cover some basics here.

The most important thing, I think, is to keep in mind the words of Henry David Thoreau when he said, "I stand in awe of my body." Consider what your body goes through during treatment for cancer. Major surgery, which is always dangerous; toxic chemotherapy, which is crazy to even think about as a voluntary action; radiation, which is so toxic the technicians can't even stay in the room with you; hormonal therapy, another variety of which may have contributed to your cancer in the first place. Any critical thinker, looking at the regimen of care for a potentially deadly disease, and knowing that you were accepting it willingly, would conclude that you need to be institutionalized! And yet we submit to it because it's what we have, and to a very large extent, it works.

One of the first things you might notice when you begin chemotherapy is dryness—dryness of everything. Skin, mouth, eyes and all the mucosal tissue in your body go dry as the desert in August. You'd naturally expect that when the treatment ended, the dryness would go away. But it doesn't happen. I am ten and eight years out of treatment, respectively, and I am still dry as dust. The great dancer, Martha Graham, said that "the body is a sacred garment", and in a philosophical sense I agree with her. In a practical sense, though, I must say that my garment suffers from permanent static electricity!

But dryer sheets are not the answer—hydration is. We are fortunate to live in a time when a wide variety of products are available to relieve these problems with dryness. They come in simple to complex compounds of every kind: cream or lotion, drop or gel, oil or mineral. They come by themselves or in other products. They come in all shapes, colors and scents, and a variety of sizes makes it easy to carry them around. But, we have to *use* them. Not long ago I was amazed to clean my bathroom cupboards and find moisturizers of every kind, none especially better than any other, that I just hadn't used enough.

So, for dry skin, I recommend two things. First, give up your daily shower. I know, that is truly a Chicken Little threat, but I'm not alone in this recommendation. Dr. Mehmet Oz of television fame says we shower way too much in this country. If you think you just can't start your day without dunking in some warm water, then don't use soap. Shocking, I know, but I promise you'll be fine, and your skin won't feel like you've been trapped in plaster of paris. Secondly, when you do use soap, make certain it is a moisturizing soap or gel. You may have had oily skin all your life, but as your post treatment life goes on, you will need to add moisture.

You'll know you have dry eyes when your vision begins to blur and you have to blink over and over again to clear them up enough to read a street sign. And you don't even want to think about passing an eye test at your local Department of Motor Vehicles until you've figured out which eye treatment works best for you. My ophthalmologist originally recommended I use Systane, a simple eye drop. As time has gone on, I've moved to GenTeal gel drops, first the formula for dry eyes and now the formula for moderate to severe dry eyes. Interestingly enough, the prescription for my glasses has changed very little over the last 20 years, and yet I have lots more trouble seeing clearly because of this dryness of the eyes. Other companies have developed and are developing products for dry eye, and you can change—after consulting with your primary care doctor—as your eyes need them. .

Part of my dry eye problem is related to the fact that I live in the country, and I have seasonal allergies all year 'round. There are anti-histamine eye drops that can be used with moisturizing eye drops, but are used not to moisturize but to protect your eyes from allergens.

When I started to think about my eyes and my allergies, it dawned on me one day that my eye problems might be at least partly related to an allergy to make-up, so I really recommend you also look into anti-histamine eye drops and think about using hypo-allergenic cosmetics. Going back to using to my eyelash curler to lift the lashes and changing to Almay hypo-allergenic mascara didn't cure my problem with blurred vision, but it sure helped!

Allergies can also make dryness of the nasal mucosa more problematic. Dryness of those tissues can lead to frequent small, but irritating, nosebleeds and even congestion. If you develop that post treatment problem, you might try Ayr saline gel. You can also use saline spray for nasal congestion or even one of those little tea pots for the nose, but you might still need something to moisturize those tissues.

You should be able to find all these products (and others, as well) in your drugstore or supermarket, and they are all available online if you like the convenience of computer shopping,

Early in the post treatment process, if you are of AARP membership age, your oncologist will very likely want you to have a bone density test, especially if you're taking a hormone- related drug like Tamoxifen or Arimidex, to see if the near total loss of estrogen is affecting your bones. I have pre-osteoporosis, which is the case with almost everyone, so if your test shows that condition, you and your team will have decisions to make.

There are a number of drugs for osteoporosis on the market, and they do make bones denser. However, my team decided not to take that option, at least so far, because those drugs also make your bones more brittle. Brittle bones, when broken, don't always break cleanly. They tend to shatter more easily. Then if you do suffer a break, treatment and healing might be more difficult and long-lasting. Another option is to supplement with calcium and vitamin D, which was the decision my doctor and I made.

Your medical team is very likely going to want you to have a colonoscopy as well. I know. Yucky. But it really isn't. I thought it was fascinating! And, if you have any polyps in there, the surgeon can snip them out right then and there and take care of it before a serious or even critical problem develops. If your colonoscopy isn't clear, they'll schedule you for another one down the line, depending on the results of that first one. In my case, I'm on what my surgeon calls "the ten year plan". So I'll have another test in just a few more years. It's not terrible, and colon cancer and all that goes with it is. They'll sedate you, so do it!

One of the major areas of concern for patients and physicians alike is the problem of Post Mastectomy Pain Syndrome (PMPS) or chronic pain after breast surgery (British Journal of Pain, v 92(2), January 31, 2005). A European study concluded that 79% of post mastectomy patients reported chronic pain more than five years after completion of therapy (European Journal of Pain, 13 (2009) 478-485). There is substantial evidence that somewhere between 15 and 60 per cent of cancer treatment survivors experience pain in the scar, pain in the axillary (armpit), and phantom pain. The pain is described variously as burning, aching, shocking, and stabbing, while numbness and feelings of pins and needles have also been reported.

I have always known that a good deal of the pain I have, which comes unbidden, and as far as I can tell unprovoked, is clearly neuropathic pain, that is, it is pain associated with the unavoidable damage to nerve tissue, especially in the axillary, during surgery. Now I know that the pain can be a result of scar tissue growing down the arm from the axillary and the ribs and up into the shoulder from the chest as a result of the mastectomy. As time has passed, this pain from scarring can become debilitating for me as the scar tissue wraps around anything it can get its tentacles on—nerves, bones, fascia, or itself. Either condition can cause severe, relatively intense pain in the axillary area or a sensation of pressure—almost but not quite cramping--that hurts all the way through your body from chest to back. That same kind of near cramping pain can occur toward the back of the axillary and down the arm. Sometimes this pain may be confused with lymphedema, but for the most part, it is a result of scarring.

You might have constant pain or intermittent pain that interferes with your activities. Or you might have some pain that is aggravated by activity, especially when your pain involves your chest and shoulder. And if, like me, you don't have continuous pain, describing your discomfort to your medical team might be difficult, but you have to try to find the words. You really mustn't just accept it or blame it on aging, because the fact is the cause of post mastectomy pain syndrome remains a mystery for the most part. The only source of pain that is clearly understood is the pain associated with neuropathy caused by the severing of nerves during surgery and the growth of scar tissue. It may be that your pain will ease as time passes, and if it does, that will be great! But in the meantime, you have to do something about it because if you don't, it will just wear you out.

So what do you do about pain? First, you talk to your doctors. Most pain can be resolved with ordinary analgesics like ibuprofen, aspirin and the like. In some situations, opioid pain medication may be necessary, but in those cases careful monitoring is necessary to make sure addiction isn't added to the pain problem. Recently, some pharmaceutical companies have started recommending selective serotonin reuptake inhibitors (SSRI) for pain. Those drugs are generally used for depression, and I have some reservations about them, but they may well be worth a closely monitored try.

Other therapies, including meditation, physical therapy, bio-feedback, homeopathy, massage, chiropractic, aromatherapy, counseling and percussive massage might help you with your pain, but patients report that those additional alternative approaches seem to help by assisting them in accommodating to the pain more than by relieving it. And accommodating to the pain shouldn't be discounted. You can keep heavy bags off your shoulders. You can open heavy doors with your non-surgical arm. You can ask for help in lifting or moving heavy objects. It's really okay to "baby" yourself when you hurt.

While surgery is clearly the cause of some pain, chemotherapy and radiation therapy can also add to problems of pain in long term cancer survivors. The peripheral neuropathy that chemo causes in fingers and toes can continue long after treatment has ended. Virtually every breast cancer patient who undergoes radiation treatment is going to earn a spot on the edge of the lobe of the lung on the side of the surgery. That spot is almost always benign and remains so, but you shouldn't forget about it entirely. You and your physician need to at least talk about the need for chest x-rays, but if there is a lung problem, your physician is likely to notice that during your routine exams. And, of course, if you still smoke, you must stop.

Radiation, like chemotherapy, causes the skin to become tender. If you suffered a radiation burn during treatment, that part of your chest may itch for years after that burn has healed, especially when you get warm. Itching can be a part of PMPS without your having had a radiation burn, though; it may just be part of the way the whole pain syndrome manifests in you, but itching is the lowest form of pain.

Obviously, you want to pay attention to your pain and other physical aspects of cancer treatment survival, and talk them over with your primary care physician. Surgeons, neurologists and oncologists all over the world are trying to understand this syndrome and figure out how to minimize and treat it, but they don't have all the answers yet. But we do have some, so you don't have to suffer in silence. Working closely with your doctor can help you find some answers to the problems of pain, and some relief is still relief.

There are other after effects on the body that develop or continue long after your treatment is completed, and I'll take those up separately in the chapters that are more specific to them. In the meantime, keep in mind the wisdom of the Buddha, Siddhartha Gautama, who taught us that "The secret of health for both mind and body is not to mourn for the past, nor to worry about the future, but to live the present moment wisely and earnestly."

C
is for Chemotherapy

Long term survivors of chemotherapy often have problems that develop during their treatment. We all expected that. But then we thought that within a reasonable time our chemo-brain and other side effects would disappear. And often, they do. But it can also happen that later, sometimes years later, we begin to experience them again. Maybe they'll feel a little different, but they're there. And you say, "I must be losing it!" Or "I feel like I did when I had chemo-brain!" And if you're the anxious type, like me, you might even think "Am I getting Alzheimer's disease or, God forbid, a metastasis to the brain?" and scare yourself silly. So I want to tell you a tale that will introduce you to post chemo after effects so that you see that you have not gone mad. Like all tales, this one will surprise you, delight you, perhaps scare you a bit, but ultimately leave you filled with hope--at least that's my goal. So the story begins:

"A TALE OF KINGS AND KNIGHTS AND DAMSELS IN DISTRESS"

Once upon a time there was a very big war. All the kings of all the nations sent their knights into battle. This was known by some as the Great War and by others as the war to end all wars, partly because some of the kings had very powerful armies and weapons the likes of which had never been seen before. One of these weapons was a vaporous gas made of sulpher which had an odor of mustard when projected toward the king's enemies, and was, therefore, called mustard gas.

Mustard gas did not win the war for any of the kings, but it caused some of their knights to die and many, many more to suffer. After the Great War ended, though it was not the war to end all wars after all, those weapons made of poisonous gas were outlawed by all the kings involved in that war. Later, however, some lesser, newer kings would use them against their enemies, causing more deaths and much more suffering.

When the great kings became aware of the suffering knights in their kingdoms, they called upon the court physicians to do whatever was necessary to bring relief to their noble subjects. As they did this work, the court physicians began to notice an interesting thing. As they performed medical workups on their patients, they saw that the white blood cells in all the mustard gas patients were lower than normal expectations. And that got the kings' physicians to thinking, which physicians, being scientists, are inclined to do.

The physicians and scientists from the various kingdoms began to talk together about what they had noticed, and they then began to wonder about it, because scientists are always wondering about things. They knew that white blood cells were fast growing cells. They also knew that cancer cells, too, were fast growing. (Cancer was a disease that had confounded all the members of every court for a long, long time, so the kings had ordered their scientists to explore every avenue that might bring promise of a cure—no matter how strange it might be.) So, understanding they were under orders to find a cure for this disease as well as to ease the suffering of the mustard gas patients, the scientists wondered if this chemical weapon could be used in another kind of war--the war on cancer. And their work began.

In time, after experimentation and testing as scientists do, the court physicians and scientists reported to their kings that they believed this so-called mustard gas could, indeed, be used to fight the disease called cancer. But, they said, it must be injected or infused directly into the bloodstream because any other form would bring about the blistering of skin and internal organs that had caused so much suffering in the brave knights.

Now the kings were concerned about the brains of their subjects, because they all valued intelligent, informed people, but the court scientists reassured them, pointing out that there is a virtual barricade between the blood stream and the brain which would always protect the brain from the poisons contained in these chemicals. This barrier was called the blood-brain barrier, or BBB. The royal scientists explained to the kings that this BBB was a permeable membrane that only allowed what the brain needed from the blood to get through to it. The kings were satisfied, and the court physicians and scientists began to use blood borne mustard gas, which they called chemotherapy (or therapeutic chemicals), to treat certain kinds of cancers, particularly breast and ovarian cancer.

This decision made the various kings' knights very happy because there was now a chance that the new treatment would save the dames and damsels in the kingdoms. And to a very large extent, the promise was fulfilled, and many thousands of the ladies of the courts and the lands lived long and happily after their treatment was completed.

All the women of the kingdoms were not entirely pleased with the treatment itself, however, because many of them became ill from side effects of these poisonous chemicals. And many of them complained about having difficulties remembering some of the knights' names, not to mention those of the court physicians and scientists (and even their own). This side-effect was so common that it soon became known as "chemo-brain", and all the dames and damsels who were in treatment would hit a memory block, and nod knowingly at one another, and whisper, "Chemo-brain!"

"To be continued"

And so it is that we who have survived the battle against cancer have actually been treated with weapons of war! It is still shocking to the old hippie peacenik in me to know that I was actually being given mustard gas derivatives to "cure" my disease! And I had 12 rounds of the stuff put directly into my bloodstream! What, I wondered, could they have been thinking?!

Well, it turns out that it's the breathing of the gas that was so deadly. It also turns out, as a result of some accidental discharges of the stuff during World War II and a study of veterans of the Iran-Iraq war who had been purposely gassed, that mustard gas damaged fast- growing human cells. Researchers, who are trained to wonder and ask questions, began to wonder whether and ask if those chemicals in mustard gas could also kill fast growing tumor cells in cancer, and the work began.

Now, all of that sounds just hideous—mustard gas! But no matter where it came from, and no matter how much like a horror story it sounds, one fact remains: Chemotherapy saves lives. It can make you feel bad. It can affect your immune system and make you vulnerable to infection. It does cause your hair to fall out. And as I will tell you in this book, it can and does cause many. many people who subject themselves to it to struggle with a variety of after effects in a variety of degrees for the rest of their lives. But with all of that, we who have been through it, and those who love and associate with us, and those who treat us, have to remember that chemotherapy, mustard gas forefathers and all, saves lives.

Chemotherapy is a systemic treatment; it goes into and through your whole system. That's why we have problems throughout our bodies after the treatment is done. There are three ways to administer chemotherapy according to the American Cancer Society:

(1) Adjuvant chemotherapy, which is what I had both times, is used after a surgical procedure has been done to remove a cancer. Some cells may be left behind that cannot be seen. Remember Dr. Erba telling me my

cancer was "systemic but not metastasized"? That's when you use adjuvant chemotherapy.

(2) Neoadjuvant chemotherapy is a process where the chemo is given before the primary cancer treatment, such as surgery or radiation. The idea here is to reduce the size of the tumor before the primary procedure because shrinking the tumor may make it easier to remove or make it easier to treat with radiation.

The American Cancer Society also tells us there are three reasons to give chemotherapy. The first, of course, is the hope of curing the cancer, although most doctors stay away from the word "cure" when they're talking about cancer. The second reason for chemo is to control the cancer; that is, to keep it from spreading and/or growing. The third reason is palliation. Chemotherapy is used in that case to relieve symptoms and improve quality of life in advanced stage cancer.

Chemotherapy is given in a sort of "cocktail" of various agents which is given as an intravenous infusion. The mix will depend on the kind of cancer you have and what the goal is for your treatment. If you really want to know all the different categories and their reasons for being, you can check out the American Cancer Society's library on the subject. For me, it's enough to know that your medical team will make many decisions concerning your treatment, and they will continually follow your progress to make sure the chemicals they've chosen are doing their best work

Now, for people who are out of the chemotherapy stage of treatment, the important thing is to know what that cocktail was. Exactly what did your medical team put together for you to help you beat this miserable disease? Did you get the Adriamycin/Cytoxan/prednisone/Atavan combination that I did, or did you get something else? Did you follow up your infusion treatment with five years of an anti-estrogen drug (like Tamoxifen) and another five years of an aromatase inhibitor (like Arimidex)? Or did you just have one and not both. In my own case, Tamoxifen had way too many side effects for me, so I went directly Arimidex. Then I stopped Arimidex during the chemo for my ovarian cancer and finished up my five year term after that was done. I tell you all this so you'll know that everything in your treatment should be tailored to your specific situation and not any other.

You want to know how many rounds of chemo you had; if you had to delay treatments because of an inability to rebuild white blood cells; and, finally, which of the drugs, if any, made you sick. If you had radiation treatments, you will want to know everything you can about them.

You'll need all that information later when after effects begin to develop, so you want to hold onto it yourself. Your physician may retire, her clinic may change its record keeping system, you might move. So, you need to have that information (along with the tumor size, lymph node involvement, and pathology results) where you can put your hands on it because you may well develop long term after effects which will be more easily treated if your doctors have that information. And the fastest and easiest way is to get it from you. Give them copies, though, not the originals. Or ask if they have the capacity to put all your information on a jump drive so that you can easily carry it with you.

Now back to our story:

"A TALE OF KINGS AND KNIGHTS
AND DAMSELS IN DISTRESS"
Part Two

Before too long, as these things go in tales, the dames and damsels were living longer and longer, and all was well with them and the knights. And the kings were all well pleased. But then, after a while, sometimes two or three or even five years after their treatment had ended, the survivors' chemo-brain seemed somehow to have returned. That seemed odd to the ladies of the kingdoms, and when told about it, even stranger to the knights, but finally the cancer survivors began to report to the court physicians and scientists that it seemed as if they were having chemo-brain without being on chemotherapy.

At first the court physicians and scientists dismissed the reports of the dames and damsels, believing that this was just a symptom of the anxiety they knew their patients experienced over the possibility of a recurrence of this awful disease, especially in the case of breast cancer which had no end time that could be considered a cure. But then so many ladies from every kingdom everywhere reported this problem that the court physicians and scientists began to talk with each other about it, and once again they began to wonder. And after wondering for some time, they began to experiment. They reported on their findings in a wide variety of scientific journals, and finally in the 11th year of the 21st century, they had a breakthrough:

In some of the dames and damsels who had treatment for cancer with the chemicals contained in the old mustard gas, the BBB could be breached after all, and it caused an after-effect of their treatment. These dames and damsels who were affected had long-term chemo-brain!

When their findings were announced, the kingdoms around the world rejoiced, for now it was clear that the kingdoms' long term surviving women were not suffering from old age or the dreaded Alzheimer's disease or new cancers. No! The dames and damsels had a particular problem that could be identified and ultimately dealt with by the court physicians and scientists. And in the meantime, the dames and damsels all over all the kingdoms who had this so-called long term chemo-brain could learn to manage it so they would never again forget their knights' names (or their own).

"To be continued"

Although new forms of targeted cancer therapy that are not cytotoxic (poisonous to fast growing cells) are being developed, most of us are still being treated with the mustard gas derivatives, including Cytoxan and Adriamycin, and hundreds of thousands of us live with the after effects of that treatment.

On October 2, 2009, The Mayo Clinic, through its Mayo Foundation for Medical Education and Research (MFMER), confirmed in "Cancer Survivors: Managing Late Effects of Cancer Treatment", that standard chemotherapy treatments for cancer can have late and long-term effects that present problems for survivors. They write, "Your cancer treatment is over, but your risk of side effects goes on. You might be surprised to know that side effects can continue after your cancer treatment or even develop several years later... not much is known about late side effects of cancer treatment ... [so you] should find out all you can ... and use this information to take control of your health."

Chemotherapy, according to MFMER, can result in long-term side effects of fatigue, menopausal symptoms, neuropathy, chemo-brain, heart failure, kidney failure, infertility and liver problems. It can cause late side effects such as cataracts, infertility, liver problems, lung disease, osteoporosis, reduced lung capacity and second primary cancers.

Let me here introduce what MFMER characterizes as potential long term side effects of radiation. Radiation therapy, according to MFMER, can cause long term side effects of fatigue and skin sensitivity and late side effects of cataracts, cavities and tooth decay, heart problems, hypothyroidism, infertility, lung disease, intestinal problems, memory problems and second primary cancers.

The third aspect of treatment, surgery, can lead to problems with scars and chronic pain and late side effects related to lymphedema, according to MFMER.

In their book, "Your Brain After Chemo: A Practical Guide to Lifting the Fog and Getting Back Your Focus", Dan Silverman, MD, PhD, and Idelle

Davidson, journalist and cancer survivor, discuss at length the most compelling and common after effect of chemotherapy: a loss of cognitive function, including a decrease in the ability to retrieve memories and words, to organize and complete tasks, and to focus, both specifically and generally. They suggest that some molecules of some of the chemotherapeutic agents are somehow passing through the blood brain barrier. They write, "The blood-brain barrier is the best defense we have to protect our brains from toxic substances…the barrier will allow in the molecules that are important for brain health [including] oxygen, glucose and amino acids…[but] the barrier rejects molecules it does not recognize or are too large or are too electrically charged…Certainly the blood brain barrier should stop most chemotherapy right at the gate. So, then, how are its toxins sneaking through?".

I asked this question of Jorg Dietrich, M.D., Ph.D., a neuro-oncologist at Harvard University, one of the original participants in the definitive study at the University of Rochester. He said the mechanism for uptake of chemo agents in the brain is still a mystery; however, they know they are there because they can be found in measurable amounts in the spinal fluid. If it's in the spinal fluid, then it is in the brain, and I'll tell you more about how that all works when we get to the chapter on Nerves.

The team at the University of Rochester and Harvard University reported an important breakthrough in 2008. In the on-line journal, "Science Daily", in an article dated April 22, 2008 they reported that they had linked a chemotherapy drug called 5-fluorouracil, or 5-FU, to central nervous system damage which could be related to memory loss "…and, in extreme cases, seizures, vision loss, and even dementia". The report goes on to say, "…these cognitive side effects [are] often dismissed as the byproduct of fatigue, depression, and anxiety related to cancer diagnosis and treatment".

More recently, Northwestern University's Feinberg School of Medicine reported in the Summer, 2011 issue of its journal, "WARDROUNDS", that a new Northwestern Medicine study shows that many cancer survivors "still suffer moderate to severe problems with pain, fatigue, sleep, memory and concentration" after treatment is completed. Associate Professor of Medicine Lynne Wagner, Ph.D. reported on the Northwestern study at the American Society of Clinical Oncology meeting held in Chicago on June 4, 2011. She said "We were surprised to see how prevalent these symptoms still are" and went on to say, "We don't have a great system to provide care to cancer survivors. Cancer survivors are left to put the pieces together to find optimal care."

The Northwestern study was quite large with a sample of 248 survivors of breast, colorectal, lung and prostate cancer, and most of the patients included in the study were more than five years beyond their diagnosis. The journal article reports that one of the study's conclusions was that "[c]ancer survivors seem to slip through the cracks in healthcare in terms of getting treatment for their pain and other symptoms" after treatment is finished.

At this point we can say we know chemotherapy can cause at least some of the problems experienced by some of us who have undergone that treatment. We know that some chemotherapeutic agents are making their way into the brain which is the likely cause of the problems, and we know the problems can last for a very a long time after treatment is completed and patients are cancer free. According to Dr. Dietrich, the agents in chemotherapy (yes, the mustard gas) cross the blood/brain barrier in somewhere between 10% and 80% of cancer patients who receive systemic chemotherapy. These agents can damage some of the millions of neurons (nerve cells) in the brain and affect neural processes in such a way as to produce what we call chemo brain as well as the other mental and physical functions that I've mentioned.

I know this might sound frightening at first, but we have to remember that the beginning of understanding the cause is also the beginning of finding the cure. As long as there is no apparent reason for our confusion and memory loss and pain and the many other things cancer treatment survivors experience, we can be overcome by anxiety. I remember being afraid I had a metastasis to the brain or Alzheimer's because I was so often confused and could not retrieve memories, and I was so relieved when I read Dr. Dietrich's 2006 journal article, I danced in my living room. I danced because when we know the things we're going through are real, then we know that somewhere there is an answer, and we can bring to our hearts the courage we need not only to manage our problems but to insist that we be heard and to push for the right treatments and ultimately a cure for us and a preventative for those who follow.

I danced because I know some of the behaviors we manifest because of our cancer treatment affect not only ourselves but those around us. Our families, friends, co-workers and virtually anyone else with whom we have a relationship are profoundly affected by our post-chemo maladies. We are not the same as we used to be, and they don't know how to handle us any more than we do. We're not as effective or efficient on the job as we used to be, and we're afraid others will notice, and they're afraid to mention it if they do! We are supposed to be well, but it looks to others like we're not willing to let go of being sick. And all of it makes us angry and ashamed. But this discovery and others that are coming could take that all away!

It's clear that we need more care, but it isn't yet broadly available to us from the scientific and medical communities. As cancer survivors, we expect to return to normal within a reasonable time after treatment ends, and our doctors expect that, too. But when we don't, we have to learn as much as we can and then take a leadership role in our own care as the Mayo Clinic article suggests. And that's the reason for this book.

Of course, the notion of brain damage or brain injury can be frightening, but an enormous amount of work is being done in this arena because of traumatic brain injury, a newly recognized interest in concussions, post-traumatic stress disorder, and other (for lack of a better word) mental disabilities. The sooner the mental and nervous issues experienced by long-term chemotherapy survivors are recognized as legitimate, the sooner the knowledge being gathered in those related areas can be applied to us. And that's a whole bunch better than thinking you've lost your mind and will never be the same again!

Okay. Now you have some science to back you up, so I can take off my professor hat. The late reporter, Hal Boyle, said "Professors simply can't discuss a thing. Habit compels them to deliver a lecture". But I don't agree. I just learned a long time ago that until we have a shared understanding of the topic at hand, we can't talk about anything in a meaningful way. But once we do have that common clarity we can have a dialogue or a discussion, and we can come to hear and use the words of the great mythologist, Joseph Campbell, who said:

> Participate joyfully
> in the sorrows of the world.
> We cannot cure the world of sorrows,
> but we can choose to live in joy.
>
> The world is perfect. It's a mess.
> It has always been a mess.
> We are not going to change it.
> Our job is to straighten out
> our own lives.

Let's begin!

D
is for Doctors

My mom had white coat syndrome. Wikipedia, the online encyclopedia, defines white coat syndrome as "a phenomenon in which patients exhibit elevated blood pressure in a clinical setting but not in other settings." Now, I know Wikipedia isn't the most reliable source in the world on all the things it covers, but this time Wiki is quoting Dr. Norman Swan who is a medical consultant for ABC News. So that's got some merit, and it fits with what I know of my mother's experience. By the time she got to Dr. Pirruccello's office (she being very fond of Dr. Pirruccello and having the greatest faith in his ability as a physician), her usually low blood pressure would be sky high. Dr. P would have to leave her alone to sit and breathe for a few minutes during each visit and then take her blood pressure again to see if he could get a proper reading. She became anxious every time she had to see any doctor, even this one she liked so much, and Dr. Pirruccello doesn't even wear a lab coat in his office!

Now, we who are cancer patients just can't afford to have "white coat syndrome" because we have not only to trust and respect all of our doctors and their staffs, but that trust and respect has to be mutual because we must feel free to ask questions of them. They, in turn, must not give us a metaphorical pat on the head and send us on our way. We need to know what's going on, and they need to give us answers. We need to know what the plan is and what we can expect as we follow the plan. Otherwise our blood pressure readings might never be accurate!

What long term survivors have to get used to, though, is that the number of people on the team shrinks as time goes by. In the first years of my two cancers I had three oncologists, one OB/GYN, two surgeons, Dr. Pirruccello and two teams of infusion nurses and techs. Recently, Dr. Alali promoted me out of cancer care. When he was first ready to move me to annual visits, I wasn't yet secure enough for that change and wanted to keep seeing him every six months. We compromised on eight months that year, and now I'm okay with having graduated. So now it's Dr. P and me, and we make a good team.

What all that means is that once you have survived the treatment, the person you will ultimately be dealing with is your primary care physician. I don't understand it at all, but I know many people who don't like their primary care physicians. When I ask them why they don't change, they really don't have an answer, but I think it's a form of "white coat syndrome" that makes them afraid of questioning what they perceive as authority. It's the same thing that keeps lots of people from asking for a second opinion (or my students from asking for help). Whatever it is, though, we who have survived cancer treatment can't afford to give into whatever emotion is driving that reluctance. One of my favorite poets, Marge Piercy, in her poem "Unlearning to not speak", addresses this reluctance to speak up as it relates to women:

"She must learn again to speak
starting with I
starting with We
starting as the infant does
with her own true hunger
and pleasure
and rage".

And we might indeed have to develop a sense of anger as we work up the courage to speak to the "white coat". But we just have to have a primary care physician who will work with us when we begin to sense that we have problems that might somehow be associated with our cancer treatment. I don't know what I would have done when I first began to feel them if I hadn't had a doctor who was as open to new ideas and willing to try to find answers as Dr. P because it's only in the last year that science is beginning to catch up with those of us who survive.

For example, the first report to the Society of Clinical Oncology of a possible solid connection between chemotherapy and central nervous system related problems was just made in July, 2011!! I'll talk lots more about that in other chapters, but the important point is that science, which we usually rely upon to guide us, is behind us in this situation, so the partnership between the primary care doc and the patient must be reciprocal. We have to be able to learn together because as patients, we only know what we feel, and no primary care physician can keep track of all the research that's coming out on this topic of long term survival because it's coming from virtually every area of the profession—oncology, neurology, radiology, hematology, and nearly all the other "ologies".

My primary care physician has never hesitated to order a test to eliminate any possible cause of any possible concern I might have. He has never once objected to my bringing material to him that I've found on the internet, and he has never once failed to pay attention to it, discuss it with me, and follow up when we decide together that a follow-up is a good idea. And he has never once suggested that my complaint might well be due to aging. Not once in more than ten years!

That's the kind of doctor you deserve and need for the long term, and I encourage you to settle for nothing less. Too much is going on in the field of long term and long lasting effects of cancer treatment for you to have anything less. But don't be getting any ideas about taking mine! Instead, give your doctor a copy of this book and see how she or he reacts. That's going to tell you a lot, and will be the beginning of your becoming a leader in this whole new aspect of the cancer fight. You can tell your guy or gal that my guy was one of the first to read this book as I dropped it by his office one or two chapters at a time. And when I showed the outline to Dr. Alali, my oncologist, he said, "Patricia, you must write this book. We need this information." (You can't have him either.)

I tend to get a bit intense on this subject of doctor/patient relationships, especially since I was recently diagnosed with Parkinson's Disease by a different doctor who offered me a prescription for "very expensive" medication that "might hold off the disease". I was livid! If he had been willing to listen to me, he would have known that the unsteady gait and the tremor in my hand, which were the basis for his diagnosis, were a result of my hip pain (I needed more vitamin D) and the extensive scar tissue in my arm, chest and shoulder. But he wasn't willing to hear me, and we won't be seeing each again. This danger of serious misdiagnosis is my greatest fear for cancer treatment survivors!

But let me calm down and leave the letter D with the gentler words of former Miss America, Mary Ann Mobley, herself a Stage III breast cancer survivor: "Have a hand in your own treatment. I have nothing but praise for our doctors, but I think they could help us better, and we can help them if we work together." That sums it up nicely.

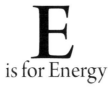

E
is for Energy

I have fond memories of energy. I used to have a real trifecta of the stuff: enthusiasm, strength and stamina! I can't begin to tell you how much I could accomplish during any given day. My home, my garden, my work, my family all benefited from my almost inexhaustible stores of energy. I was totally in sync with Secretary of State Colin Powell, who said, "The chief condition on which, life, health and vigor depend, is action. It is by action that an organism develops its faculties, increases its energy, and attains the fulfillment of its destiny." Even after my first round of cancer treatment I could go at a better than steady pace for hours on end.

But I lost it.

I didn't lose all my energy at once. After my first cancer treatment my energy levels returned to normal pretty quickly. In fact, I taught all through that treatment, and in those days before all the budget cuts we have to deal with now, that was nine hours a week in the classroom as well as the grading of papers and all the rest that goes into teaching. I used to walk 30 minutes a day, usually on my treadmill, so I could get my continuing education requirements out of the way by watching video courses. I worked in the yard as I always had—weeding, planting, transplanting when I made an error in my design, and hauling pruned material off for recycling. I shopped and cooked for my mom and me, and just did everything a healthy woman does. I was like the line in Marge Piercy's poem *The butt of winter*, in which she writes,

> Stretch out your hand,
> stretch out your hand and look:
> each finger is a snake of energy

We even found my soccer ball-sized ovarian tumor because all the weight I was losing revealed a disturbingly large belly! And, of course, that turned out to be cancer, too, and when the surgery was healed, my little hummingbird wings churned me back into chemotherapy.

By then we had a new oncologist on staff at our hospital, Dr. Alborz Alali, so I was able to do the second round of chemo without having to drive 30 miles. And that was a good thing, because the second round of chemo was much more difficult for me. I maintained my course work at the college, but only with the help of one of my sisters who stood in for me on the days when I just couldn't do it. My white cell count dropped three times during this round, which it hadn't done the first time, and I often fell asleep during the infusions, which were being done this time through a port that Dr. Erba had placed below my collar bone.

I spent a lot more time in bed or lying on the couch, I often needed help with the shopping, and we began to have more frozen meals and take home feasts. My mom gave up her driver's license at age 90, and I worried about her in the kitchen since she had fallen while frying chicken a few years before and burned herself badly. Mother could still do the laundry, though, so I didn't have to worry about that, but I had to hire a house-keeper because I wasn't strong enough to keep up with those chores, and I had to turn more of the yard work over to my gardener. And, of course, even though I was very close to home for this series, I still had to have my daughter and my niece come in from out of town to make sure I didn't endanger anyone who might be out and about on my chemo day!. So the second round of chemo was exhausting and stressful, and a financial bur-den, as well as demanding on other people to give me more help in caring for both my mother and me.

Finally, after treatment four of the scheduled six rounds of chemotherapy, I told Dr. Alali I couldn't go on. I can see myself, my daughter at my side, my head on his desk, saying to that good doctor, "I can't do it anymore. I just can't take any more of this." And I remember just as clearly, his saying very softly, "Yes, you can. There's only a little bit more. I know you can do it". I'll never forget how done in I was and how totally supportive he was. If I hadn't liked and respected him before (which I certainly had), he'd have won me over that day. And because of his support and his belief in me and my ability to go on, I did.

I thought, of course, that once I recovered from the chemo treatments, I'd be back to normal in terms of my energy levels. I didn't have to have radiation the second time, so I was confident that my energy would re-turn rather quickly, and it did. I got back into all my courses, joined a gym (which I loved), returned to my yard work, and we got to eat real food again. I have to admit I kept the housekeeper, though! She not only helped me, but my mom enjoyed her company. So, I was back to normal and happy to be there.

A couple of years later my nearly 95 year old mother's heart condition began to worsen, and she began to need a great deal more of my time and energy. Just being with her as she experienced heart attacks that gradually worsened sapped my strength as I knew she was in pain and didn't want me to do anything about it. All I could do was hold my breath and wait it out with her. So, of course, that whole period, which lasted about eight to ten months became more and more exhausting as the weeks passed by.

After my mother died, just a few days before that 95th birthday, I never did regain my strength. And as time has passed over these last five years, I have lost more and more of it. You'll recall that two to five years is the time when reports of post treatment after effects begin to kick in, and it had been three years since my ovarian cancer diagnosis when my mom passed, so I was right on target.

When people talk about energy depletion after cancer treatment, they refer to it is "fatigue". But that's not even close. This stuff that hits long term chemotherapy survivors is even worse than Chronic Fatigue Syndrome!

We know that fatigue can be a good thing. As the poet writes, fatigue can even be "sweet". You can feel fatigued at the end of a good day's work and at the same time feel great. You can look at or think about the things you accomplished to earn that fatigue and feel fantastic about yourself and your accomplishments. I remember how lovely it was just a few years ago to sit in my garden at the end of a long day of work and sip a glass of wine while I admired the results of my efforts. It's as Ken Kesey, one of my favorite authors, said, "There's something about taking a plow and breaking new ground. It gives you energy", and that's true even when you do it on a smaller scale than a plow, say with a rototiller or even a garden fork! So I'm something of a fan of fatigue, and I miss it as much as I miss energy.

So while I was really very clear about what this I have to deal with now isn't, it took a lot of time and thought to come up with what this really is. I looked up lots of words that I thought might work, like "inertia" and "sluggish", but they all indicate laziness, an unwillingness to move. Finally, I realized that I can only explain it by way of a metaphor: This long out of chemotherapy, I have become a cell phone! Some days I wake up, and I have no bars!

When your cell phone has no bars, you can't do anything with it, and when my body has "no bars", the problem is the same. And, as with the cell phone, the only thing I can do is recharge the battery. The problem here is that when I charge the cell phone, I plug the thing in and go about my business until it's done its thing. Or I can even plug it into the dashboard of my car and let it charge away while I do my errands. But the only way to get some bars back in me is to lay my body down and sleep. And that is not always convenient. And it is rarely what I want to do.

And before I understood how this thing works, while I was still operating on the notion of "fatigue" and not "no bars available", I would just hop out of bed and start on my day, going full speed ahead at whatever might be on my list. And then in a few hours I would sit down to have a little lunch, take a little break, only to find myself waking up from an unexpected bout of recharging (most people call that taking a nap) two or three hours later. I would be so surprised because I hadn't felt sleepy or even drowsy. I hadn't felt "tired" or "fatigued". I had been fine. Just sat down for a half hour lunch break and out like the proverbial light. The fatigue I experience is exactly as described by Pardini, et al, which is to say, "…an overwhelming lack of physical or mental energy". And Dr. Glen Johnson, in his e-book on traumatic brain injury, compares mental fatigue to a car that runs out of gas, saying "… it's as if the brain runs out of chemicals and just shuts down".

But I found out that I was far from being alone in this sometimes debilitating after-effect as it is the single most prevalent complaint of long-term cancer treatment survivors. But to tell you about that I have to put on my academic costume again and become a bit professorial so we will all understand what's been going on in this area of post-chemotherapy survival. So, here we go again with the scientists.

In 2002 Servais, et al, at the University Medical Centre, Nijmegen, The Netherlands did a study on fatigue in 150 disease-free breast cancer treatment survivors as a quality of life issue, and found that fatigue was reported as a problem "long after curative treatment for cancer has ended" and "38% of the of the sample were severely fatigued, compared with 11% in a matched sample of women without a history of cancer." In 2006, Bower, et al, investigated 763 breast cancer survivors for post-treatment fatigue, and found that approximately 34% of the women who participated in their study "… reported significant fatigue at 5-10 years after diagnosis.

So that means in both those studies, more than a third of the long-term cancer survivors were reporting fatigue as a major quality of life issue. Neither of those studies was able to relate the fatigue problem specifically to cancer treatment and concluded that it must be caused by a combination of factors, including "depression [primarily], pain, sleep disturbance, comorbid medical conditions and age."

By 2004, however, da Jong, et al, of the University Hospital Maastricht. The Netherlands, and School of Nursing and Faculty of Medicine, American

University of Beirut, Beirut, Lebanon, were able to report that there was a connection between fatigue and doxorubicin (known to us as Adriamycin), cyclophosphamide (known to us as Cytoxan), methotrexate and 5-fluorouacil (CMF) which is also called 5-FU. That's the cocktail used in adjuvant chemotherapy for breast and many other cancers. They said, "Partly as a result of longer cancer survival, it is increasingly being realised that quality of life in cancer patients is affected by fatigue. The National Comprehensive Cancer Network (NCCN) stated that fatigue affects 70-100% of cancer patients." They also reported that fatigue was more prevalent and intense in those participants who had had mastectomies as opposed to lumpectomies and in those who also had radiation as opposed to those who did not. And, they said, that patients in their "doxorubicin group, involving five different therapies, and those in their CMF group respectively experienced "direct increase in fatigue" and a "moderate direct increase in fatigue".

Most recently, in July, 2011, a research team at the University of Rochester Medical Center in New York and the Harvard Medical School reported on the conclusion of their long term study on how chemotherapy might affect the brain, and they established a direct link between that chemotherapy drug I mentioned before, 5-fluorouracil (5FU or CMF) and the central nervous system, which controls brain function which affects the occurrence and intensity of fatigue, among other things.

My cap and gown are back on their hangars now, so let me just say it's a relief to me to know that some folks know some things about what might be causing this awful after effect of chemotherapy, and it's a relief to know that I was right about my experience of terrible fatigue as being related to my own chemotherapy. I know how I was before, and I'm not that way anymore.

But back to my cell phone analogy, fatigue is measured at the end of the day after the job or jobs are done. Now I awake every morning and ask myself how many "bars" I have as a result of charging my batteries with sleep. Sometimes I wake up with a full five bars! That's always an exciting experience, a fabulous feeling. It's like Marge Piercy—yes, again—writes in her poem, *The window of the woman burning*, "Woman you are the demon of a fountain of energy". How I love those days!

So the question is: How do we get more of those "demon" days? Well, it's not easy, first because we women tend to make almost everything a job of work. When you have long term chemo-brain, you just can't afford to do that. But there are lots of things you can do.

The first thing you want to do is ask your doctor to run blood tests to rule out problems with your thyroid, anemia, low blood sugar or the complex condition called Chronic Fatigue Syndrome. When those are out of the way, then you can take over, but that means lots of changes in the way you do things. Years ago, whenever one of us was facing a big organizational problem, we would quote an old Texas lawyer, whose name I've forgotten, and we would say to each other: "Begin…The rest is easy". Well, that might be true if all you're going to do is install a new computer system, but if you're going to change the way you live your life, it's a little more difficult, mostly because you're going to have to begin and begin again and begin yet again before you and the people around you find and adapt to what works for you. But let me give you some suggestions that can get you started.

Obviously, the best idea is to try to not get to the "no cell bar" stage in the first place. So some simple ideas that may help with that goal involve (wouldn't you just know) stress reduction! A Canadian researcher named Hans Selye came to an understanding of human biological stress. Selye called his discovery general adaptation syndrome (GAS). Basically, Selye said we respond to stressors by releasing hormones that result in the well-known "fight or flight" response. He says that after the stressful event, we need time to settle down and reabsorb those leftover chemical responses to the thing that endangered us. Then, he said, if we don't have that time for recovery, we stay in a state of arousal. Then, another stressor comes along, and our bodies respond by sending out those chemical warnings, and our stress level goes a bit higher. At that point we need even more time to recover, but in our busy lives we don't get it, and before long we are constantly in an advanced state of stress caused by our own chemistry! Combine that with our tendency to take on too much and make everything a job, and you have a recipe for fatigue. If you do it long enough, your eyes will open one morning and you will find you have no cell bars and can't get out of bed.

Now you can see how that happens to all of us all the time. Think about the "mental health days" we all take from work. For the most part, those are a result of the body saying NO MORE! to stress. Imagine, then if you are a cancer survivor. Most of us leave treatment with Post-Traumatic Stress Disorder to begin with. Then, over time, if we develop neurological and cognitive symptoms because of chemotherapy having breached the blood-brain barrier, we may be even more susceptible to General Adaptation Syndrome, and end up with no bars much more quickly and much more easily than people who have never been through cancer treatment.

So, let's begin with a simple little item: the to-do list! We all have a to-do list, whether it's written down or carried around in our heads. I recommend that you write down everything you have to do-- at home, at work, with your family, everything—for the next week. Now, look at the list very carefully and begin to ask these questions about each item:

(1) Does it HAVE to be DONE? We fill our days with lots of things that don't really have to be done, and for the most part, we don't do them. But we still carry them around on the to-do list and berate ourselves for every day that we don't get them done, which, of course, makes them more stressful. And they aren't even the necessary items! But let's say an item does have to be done. Then your next step is

(2) Does it have to be done BY ME? I cannot begin to tell you the number of adults I have in my classes, many of them single moms, who are going to college, working full time and are still making their kids' beds and cleaning their rooms! What's with that? What needs to be done here is some delegating! Put those kids (and their father if he's around) to work! If you are long term cancer treatment survivor, and you're trying to do this super-mom thing, you're going to have more no cell bar days than you can imagine.

That will affect your health, first of all, and then your job, your grades, your emotional well-being, and ultimately the quality of life for everyone around you. Finally, if there are still items on your to-do list after stripping away the unnecessary and delegating as much as you can, your next step is

(3) Does it have to be done TODAY? Realistically, you will only do today what you know deep inside has to be done today. You might worry about the other things, and you might complain about how difficult it all is and how busy you are, but you'll only accomplish what you know you need to accomplish on a given day. And within that framework, you'll do the things you like best first, and push all the other stuff to the end of the day, where it might well leave you in a state of collapse as it conflicts with other things on your list.

Now I can promise you that my method really does work, but only if you are brutally honest with yourself, and that might take some time. All habits are hard to change, but this one affects our self-image, that whole super-mom thing, and that can be hard to handle. "I can't" are two really bad words in most women's minds, but you have to get over that to avoid being too exhausted to do anything. This whole to-do list conflict can be described in the words of motivational speaker, Dale Carnegie, who said "Our fatigue is often caused not by work, but by worry, frustration and resentment".

The next piece of advice I have for you is that you go to bed at the same time every night and plan on getting seven to eight hours of sleep. I know that's hard to do, but that's why you have to handle the to-do list first! I go to bed at 9:00 every night, read until 10:00 and get up at 6:30 in the morning on the days that I work. On free days, I sleep until 7:00 or 7:30. I don't have a television set in my bedroom. Television is stimulating because of sound, color and the quick changes of scene editors make to keep us interested in their program. If you're interested in the program, you're not going to go to sleep, and if you are a long term cancer survivor, you need your sleep. Take this advice from Benjamin Franklin, who said "Fatigue is the best pillow", and go to bed!

There are more steps that you can take to try to deal with this failure of energy problem. Before this problem developed in my life I rarely indulged in caffeine, but now I find that a cup or coffee, green tea, or a cappuccino in the morning, helps pick me up a little. I wouldn't want to overdo that because the stimulative properties of caffeine could well interfere with sleep. But another cup early in the afternoon could be helpful as well. Those high-energy drinks that my students slam down are not a good idea for us at all (or them, for that matter). Ironically, you have to be careful with alcohol, too, although alcohol is a depressant. The after effects of chemotherapy may well change the way you respond to alcohol. Exercise also helps, and a short nap, say 20 minutes or so, can help quite a lot if you have the time and a place to do that during the day. But if you get to the place where you're taking two or three hour naps every day, then it's time to start working on the problem with your doctor.

Finally, there is medication. As I showed you at the beginning of this conversation, physicians tended to think this debilitating fatigue was related to depression and anxiety—as someone said, we were making "a career" of our cancer. So, they prescribed anti-depressants and selective serotonin reuptake inhibitors (SSRI) to see if they would help. Over time I have found that the SSRI can work well for me in getting through especially difficult times, so I do occasionally take a short series of that medication if we decide it might be helpful. We watch it very carefully and stop it as soon as it's done what we want it to do.

Other medications, such as those used to treat Attention Deficit Disorder and Attention Deficit Hyperactivity Disorder, are sometimes considered. I would not be willing to take those myself, but I wouldn't discourage anyone from looking into them depending on the severity of their problem. My problem with those medications is that they are so closely related to amphetamines, and there is no substantial evidence that those conditions actually exist. Dr. Phil of television fame has said that 70% of the cases of ADD and ADHD in children today are incorrect diagnoses. Especially knowing now that it is possible that a large number of people who have survived treatment with doxyrubicin and cytotoxan for cancer may have nervous system damage due to a breaching of the blood-brain barrier, we must be especially careful about stimulating the nervous system since we cannot know how medication will affect the neural pathways and synapses in the brain.

But you must do what you can until the researchers make more progress in determining specific areas of the brain that might be affected which may well lead to specific medications to help us. Similar work is being done in an effort to help other groups who suffer from episodes of an "overwhelming lack of physical or mental energy". And in the meantime, you just can't "run yourself ragged", which was a favorite piece of advice from my mom back in the days when I had that virtual trifecta of energy—just like hummingbirds.

I do know that all of us who suffer from this debilitating exhaustion can surely relate to the words of actress, Patricia Richardson, who said about her life, "The truth is, I've been going pretty much nuts all year. I constantly have to fight being scattered. I feel like I'm on automatic pilot from fatigue. The hardest thing is trying to be present, living for the moment, for everybody in the family". But if we want our long term survival to continue, we have to find ways to avoid the state that so overwhelmed Ms. Richardson.

F

is for Food

I come from a big family that started when my mother married a dashing young college basketball player who took her home with him to Oregon to live and work in his grandmother's boarding house. My mom also grew up in a big family, enjoying a pretty carefree life with lots of adults around to handle the work of running a home. When she arrived at my great-grandmother's boarding house and found she was expected to help prepare and serve two meals a day, six days a week, and one on Sunday for 15 people, including the family members, it was quite a shock to her! In making the adjustment to this new demanding life style my mother learned a lot about hard work, but most of all, she learned to cook, and she learned it well.

So, by the time my mom had four children, was widowed and married my step-father with his two children she knew how to feed a table full. Her menus, in the style of the day, were built on the basics: meat, starch (potatoes or noodles), something green, bread, something to drink and dessert. Being raised in the 50's wasn't "Leave it to Beaver" but it was a time when people still ate vegetables from their gardens and fruit from their trees. The average backyard provided many of the basics for good eating. It wasn't until the 60s that we began to move our diets towards prepared, packaged, frozen, and fast foods.

As I grew up and had my own family, my mother's philosophy of food went with me. Meat, starch, something green, a proper drink, bread and dessert were our staples. When I began to work full time my family began to eat out more often, and we lost many of the eating patterns that we had been brought up with. Society had changed and so had I.

But then, of course, cancer arrived, and my whole idea of food changed dramatically. The first thing I had in my mind was the advice of one of my parents' friends who had had cancer. She said if I ever had to have chemotherapy, I should eat and eat and eat to keep myself from getting sick. That's what she had done, and she had outlived her prognosis by many months, so I figured that was good advice. Then I found the National Institutes of Health booklet on how to eat during chemotherapy, and that was very helpful because while it also said eat whatever you can whenever you can, it gave some powerful advice about eating on chemo day. I remember it said I'd feel really good on the first day because of the additives in the chemo cocktail. It said I would want to eat, and I would want to eat a good, full meal. And then it said I shouldn't give into that desire. It said nothing hot, nothing spicy, nothing too filling on that first day. So I followed those two pieces of advice, and I was never sick. However, and that is a big "however", I did gain weight for the first time in my life. The pounds just seemed to pile on, and there didn't seem to be anything I could do to help it. Everything I had learned about how to cook and how to eat had left my consciousness, leaving me muffins and milkshakes and pie and especially ice cream.

Now, I have to really work on food all the time. (Sometimes it feels like Mark Twain was right when he said, "The only way to keep your health is to eat what you don't want, drink what you don't like, and do what you'd rather not.") I know the diet for a cancer treatment survivor is high protein, low fat and complex carbohydrates. But a lot of our food today isn't good for us. Fish is excellent for cancer survivors, BUT the fish must be wild caught and fresh. Farm raised fish are fed carcinogens to make them grow bigger, faster. So I avoid those entirely and wait patiently for the salmon season to arrive.

Virtually all of our beef and poultry supplies are contaminated with hormones that can be very dangerous for us, as well as antibiotics which can result in our becoming resistant to the antibiotics that we're consuming in our food. Again, the reason for these additives is to make the animals fatter for market sooner. Our collective awareness regarding chemicals in food is on the upswing, but as cancer survivors we need to push ourselves to stay ahead of the game when it comes to food information and our health. It is encouraging to note that the Food and Drug Administration just recently ordered beef producers to stop using a particular antibiotic in cattle that is a last ditch for potentially deadly infections in humans, so that humans would not become resistant to it. Nonetheless, we can't afford to wait for decisions from the Food and Drug Administration but must put food information at the head of our list when it comes to maintaining our health. Simply stated, chemical methods used in growing and producing our foods need to be questioned. (There's a film entitled "Food, Inc", which is very revealing about this aspect of food.)

Good basic guidelines for shopping are organic, farmer's markets and fresh. Know where your food comes from and what chemicals are involved. An important area for us to look at is dairy products. Many of them contain hormones and antibiotics that have been given to the animals. We have to be careful to only buy milk and other dairy items that state in big letters that they come from cows that are not treated with hormones.

The use of pesticides and fertilizers on field crops has long been a concern and is a problem for cancer survivors. Several of these have been outlawed, but there are still plenty of them in fields all across the country.

So, try to buy organic meat, chicken, milk, eggs and vegetables whenever you can. More and more grocery stores are offering organic foods, and those that you can buy in bulk, like steel cut oatmeal, nuts, and grains tend to be easier on the budget because you can buy only as much as you need.

Being one of the many thousands of single women who has survived cancer, I want to talk a bit about how food can be managed when there's just you. Cooking for one isn't much fun, but you can make it a whole lot better. I try to get the necessary elements—protein and complex carbs with little or no fat-- into my diet throughout the day as opposed in every meal. So I have my choice of oat cereal, fruit or yogurt for breakfast, peanut butter or egg with fruit and milk for lunch, and meat or fowl or beans with salad for dinner. I also frequently make protein drinks with yogurt and fruit, and I'm never without a high protein energy bar wherever I go.

Since my most recent dental reconstruction is not yet complete, I have to focus on food that is easily chewed and not abrasive. Some weekends I cook big kettles of soup or big dishes of some of my favorite family recipes, and I have a serving or two and then freeze the rest. That definitely helps keep my food life interesting because I miss those dishes Mother used to make. And when I do that, I follow this advice from the old time comedian, W.C. Fields: "I cook with wine; sometimes I even add it to the food".

I think the biggest thing I've discovered is that the common, ordinary sandwich can be your best friend. Since I try to be very careful of portion size, I often make open face sandwiches so that I can keep the amount of bread I eat under control. You can make peanut butter, peanut butter and jelly, egg salad, egg and olive, grilled cheese or tuna sandwiches, and meet the requirements of your post-treatment diet. I buy solid core canned alba-core tuna because it seems to be healthy, at least at this point, and I eat lots and lots of canned beans. Of course, George Orwell said "We may find in the long run that tinned food is a deadlier weapon than the machine-gun". With all the talk these days about BPA in plastic and now cans, we have to wonder if the famous futurist was right! But in any case, if you add rice to beans, you have a perfect fat-free protein that doesn't cost nearly as much as a steak. And you can eat an egg or two a week unless your cholesterol levels absolutely don't allow it. Check with your doctor, though, because while recent research indicates eggs might not be so much a cause of high cholesterol as we previously thought, you and your doctor know what's best for you!

My "something green" tends to be salad, and I've learned that you can do so many good things with salads. And, of course, if you're vegan or vegetarian you have to work really hard to get the protein you need. It's probably an old saying for you green eaters, but I chuckled when I learned that George Bernard Shaw said, "Animals are my friends... and I don't eat my friends". The other piece of advice from the vegan community is "never eat anything that has a face", but if you are vegetarian or vegan you absolutely must ask your doctor for a referral to a nutritionist so you can get the protein you need.

But getting back to salads, let me recommend that you think about mixing fruit with salad greens. Some companies are even putting those combinations in bag salads these days. I like to put mandarin orange slices with butter lettuce and raspberry dressing. It's beautiful to look at and even better to eat. Another combination I like is raw spinach with either strawberries or pears. Pears also go well with a mix of spring greens. If you can begin to move away from the standard lettuce and tomato salad with ranch dressing, you can really perk up your diet, and if you make a big fruit and green salad, with a few nuts and maybe some small chunks of jack or Monterey cheese, and a bit of chopped egg, you'll have a full meal that's tasty, filling and good for you.

You can certainly have pasta every week or so. It should be whole wheat pasta, and the sauce should be a simple red sauce. You can add browned, well drained ground meat to the red sauce if you like, but be sure to drain that fat off. I love Alfredo sauce, but it's a little fatty, and I have yet to find a low-fat brand that isn't also low in flavor. Bread, of course, should be whole grain— always.

For dessert, nothing beats fresh fruit or melon. Here's a hint about fresh fruit. You know that when you buy fruit in the stores, if you don't have a farmer's market nearby, it is not ready-to-eat ripe. So, save a shoe box, put the fruit in the shoe box and put the fruit filled shoe box in your laundry room. Give it a couple of days and the juice will drip from your fingers and your chin! Obviously, when you do this, you don't want to buy more than you can eat before your next trip to the store or else it gets too ripe and goes to waste.

Be careful to avoid grapefruit and grapefruit juice unless you verify with your doctor that it will not increase the dosage strength of any medication you are taking!

On special occasions I like a fresh fruit tart that's so easy to make if you use refrigerated pie crust. If you absolutely have to, you can even use frozen fruit to make a tart. Another special dessert that I make for family occasions is a pear cake, made in a spring pan in the manner of upside-down cake, but with Bosc pears which are firm enough to hold up during baking. Top that with a little organic whipped cream, and you and your guests will be in heaven. Either one of those, by the way, can be a breakfast treat or something special for brunch.

And then, of course, there is chocolate. Chocolate is just a killer temptation for me (and I think most of us). So here's my advice. You can have all the chocolate you want as long as you eat it exactly as my aunt, who has Type II diabetes, does. She has one piece of chocolate every Sunday evening for dessert! Just one piece, once a week. If you're strong enough to only have a bit of the forbidden every week, you should be okay!

Bon apétit!

G
is for General Health

I n her classic novel "Jane Eyre", Charlotte Bronte has her heroine in a discussion with the local priest about what it takes for little girls to avoid the eternal fires of hell. Jane answers all the pastor's questions properly and respectfully, and when he asks specifically, "And what must you do to avoid it?" she replies, "I must keep in good health and not die." She reports that the priest found her answer unacceptable. I suppose it might well be so from the perspective of the local religious leader, but for those of us who have survived cancer and its treatment, there is no better advice.

When we spend a year or more dealing with one, and really only one, health issue, we tend to forget that there are some routine medical and dental procedures that we need to take care of. It's kind of the idea of out of chemo, out of radiation, done with medicine. But, of course, that isn't true. The number of books on health, fitness and medicine and the number of doctors on television and the Internet show us that. But we probably should listen again to Mark Twain who offered this up for our consideration (and a chuckle): "Be careful about reading health books. You may die of a misprint". I promise that won't happen with this book.

With regard to our cancer, we need to see our oncologist at least every six months for a couple of years, and we need to see our primary care physicians at least that often. I say this despite the fact that Plato, one of my helpful philosophers, wrote "Attention to health is life's greatest hindrance". I don't disagree with Plato on many things, but we're miles apart on this one. But then, medicine has made enormous strides in the last 2,500 years or so!

Soon after my treatment for my first cancer ended, my oncologist wanted me to have a bone density test and a colonoscopy. She wanted to get a baseline reading on both those parts of me, and I'm happy to say that I am pre-osteoporotic, and I'm on the ten year plan for a follow up colonoscopy. It's surprising to me how good it feels to get good results on ordinary tests that everyone else takes. It seems so normal.

I have a spot on my right lung which is related to radiation, and we did a chest x-ray every year for three years to make sure that spot was not changing. We also did basic tests on the vital organs that the Mayo Clinic refers to. We did a full respiratory exam, and we did a stress test to check my heart function. I imagine that when the ten year limit on the colonoscopy expires, we will also repeat those heart and lung function tests, and we may add an annual EKG to monitor my heart more closely since long term cancer treatment related heart failure shows no symptoms.

I have a mammogram every year, and for the first several years that I was out of treatment, we also did annual CT scans to ascertain if there had been any recurrence of my cancer outside the breast. There is no five or ten year "cured" period for breast cancer, so for several years we were extremely careful. Finally, about three years ago, my second oncologist said we didn't need to do any more CT scans. As he pointed out, I've had all the radiation I need!

In terms of monitoring for new cancers, I saw both oncologists every six months for seven years, and I now see my local oncologist every year. I wasn't quite ready to go to annual visits when I was first supposed to, so for a couple of years we compromised on eight months!. And now I am released from their care.

I see Dr. P every six months, in May and November, and sometimes several times in between, depending on how my fatigue, pain, and allergies are behaving. We have a regular routine. I have a small node on my thyroid gland, and we look at that and biopsy it if necessary in November. Then in May we do a basic physical with lab work to check my thyroid, my cholesterol levels and all the other things all those tubes of blood reveal. We check my medications, which, thankfully, are very few, and the supplements I take. I have taken the calcium and vitamin D I mentioned in the first chapter for years, and then as my research began to reveal the potential for nerve damage we added vitamin B. I get a flu shot every year, and, of course, every time I see any of these medical people, they check my weight (!) and take my blood pressure. A new bit of information is that we now have a vaccine for the terrible condition called shingles. If you are actively engaged in chemotherapy, you won't be allowed to have the shingles vaccine. But if you have completed your chemo, there's no reason why you shouldn't have it and eliminate your chances of getting that miserable disease. I've had the shot with no negative consequences.

We who have survived cancer cannot forget our routine health maintenance. Siddhartha Gautama, the Buddha, tells us that "The secret of health for both mind and body is…to live the present moment wisely and earnestly". And the first task in that job is to take care of our general health.

H
is for Hair

My grandmother had a way with words. They weren't always kind words, but they were on the spot. For example, she said about me from the time I was a little girl that if I'd had one more hair I'd have been a yellow dog! I don't recall taking offense at that, probably because even at a very young age I could see the near analogy. And I could feel it every morning as my mother combed out my long, fly-away fine locks and turned them—with me complaining about tangles every step of the way—into pigtails! I did take offense at that because my mother had long, fine, fly-away hair that had to be woven to hold it in place, but hers were called French braids. Anyone could see, even at three years old, that French braids must be more delicious than pigtails!

Then when I was in high school and we set our hair in a single row of pin curls to make a 50's flip, I always had a couple of pin curls left over. I had the same problem when we used hard plastic or sharp, sticky brush rollers (and actually slept on them!) to get that lovely bouffant look. We call that "big hair" today, and I was really good at big hair once I found a spot for the leftover rollers that wouldn't destroy the whole look.

Hair dryers and hot irons were a blessing. All they required was enough time to get through the mess of hair that grew and grew from my head, no matter what I did to it. And I did everything to it a person could do. I dyed it, bleached it, and permed it both at home and in salons. I was like Hillary Clinton, who said, "I'm undaunted in my quest to amuse myself by constantly changing my hair." With all that hair, I figured if what I did took some away, there would always be more. I could never have imagined that it wouldn't always be there.

Of course, I knew when I went into the first round of chemotherapy that I would lose my hair. The UCD Cancer Center nurses pulled no punches about that. And I wasn't a bit worried about it. I did read in a National Institutes of Health booklet that during chemotherapy the hair doesn't fall out all at once. You don't wake up one morning and find your locks laid out neatly on your pillow. Oh, no, it said. Your hair will come out in clumps, it said. It will come out in clumps over a period of days or weeks, it said. Well, I wasn't having any of that because all I could imagine was that I'd be whipping up a big batch of cabbage rolls (my specialty) for my family, and a big bunch of hair would fall into the kettle. So, I shaved my head.

Being bare-headed was a very strange experience for me after nearly 60 years of all that focus on all that hair. But I have a pretty good shape to my head, and I thought with big hoop earrings and a lot of imagination I kind of resembled a short, white version of the beautiful Black model, Imam. I quoted the famous Stoic philosopher, Seneca, who said, "I don't consider myself bald, I'm just taller than my hair". (Those ancient Roman Stoics can be a big help in more things than you could ever imagine.)

For public appearances, like in my classroom, I wore little bandana caps that I made out of quilting squares, and I had a whole wardrobe of them, so that was no problem. I bought a night cap from the American Cancer Society and put that to good use because I was totally surprised to find out how cold you can get through a long winter's night when your head is bare!

But the real surprise came quite a bit later. Before I went into my first round of chemotherapy I had read in several publications that perhaps the worst possible thing about chemo was the loss of one's hair. I scoffed. "How silly" I thought. It's just hair. It'll grow back. And it did—sort of. But I was still in my caps for going outside the house when the second round of chemo was scheduled. So I shaved my head again (not a very time-consuming process this time) and began "infusing" again. The second time around I was much less conscious of my bare dome until a neighbor came to the door and, not giving it a thought, I answered without covering up. The astonished look on his face taught me that while I had become pretty comfortable with having no hair, that wasn't the case for everyone.

So, the second round of chemo ended, and I sat back and waited for my hair to come in. A friend of mine who had gone into therapy after me was out and had so much thick, curly hair she couldn't get a comb through it. I didn't expect curls, but I was looking forward to thick again.

The first sprouts were pretty exciting to see, although there seemed to me to be a lot of scalp between them. But I assured myself that it was a process. Nobody had ever said I was born with all that hair my grandmother loved to comment on but hated to comb. Patience, I said to myself. You'll be back to amusing yourself with it again in no time.

But I was wrong. My hair did not even really begin to come back until almost nine years after the completion of the first rounds of chemotherapy. As I write this it's still coming in, but now it's thick enough all over to hide my very pink scalp, and I don't have to worry about scaring students away. (The first time I went to class uncovered, pretty sure I had enough hair to get by, I arrived early. The look on the face of the first student to arrive, told me a lot. "Not yet, huh", I said to Isaac, and all he could do was slowly shake his head, "no".)

You might well ask why it took so long to get my former full head of hair growing again. I know I did. I asked doctors and hair dressers and did my research. I begged for an answer, and my respondents seemed to have one of two possibilities available: (1) I don't know, or (2) Well, all of us begin to lose our hair as we age. There it was again, that age thing, and I wasn't buying it. I was the girl who might have been a yellow dog but for one more hair, and now people were telling me I would be half bald forever? That answer just wasn't good enough, especially since it seemed to be the one I got for every post-treatment problem I had.

So, I kept working on finding an answer, and in the meantime I tried the wigs I'd purchased for special occasions during the first round of treatment, but all of them were still too tight and way too hot. When I got enough hair to hold onto them I invested in some hair pieces, but they had to have clasp closures because combs just fell out, taking the pony tail or twist or chignon with them, often at the most inopportune times. Wigs were tight and hot and hairpieces were heavy and not quite my shade, and way more attention was being paid to my not having hair than had ever been paid to all the hair I once had.

One day, not so very long ago, I went to have my hair cut. As my friend, Jean, worked and worked on the back of my very short "do", she said, "I don't know what I'm going to do with all these cowlicks!" I couldn't understand what she was saying. I never had more than one cowlick on the crown of my head and one in my hairline. But she assured me I had them all over the back of my head and finally showed me what she was seeing by giving me a hand mirror and twirling the chair around. The back of my head looked like a pinwheel!! The short strands of hair swirled out from the center of my large, pink head. I was stunned.

By this time I had been using a product line called Nioxin, which I highly recommend, and my hair had begun to grow a bit thicker. I could tell when hair was finally poking through because my scalp would itch when I applied the shampoo. I had noticed that as new hair came in, it tended to force its way through and push the existing hair out of the way. But this pinwheel effect was new and definitely not a style anyone would want to voluntarily adopt. Something had to be done! So Jean forced the hair on the back of my head down, added a good bit of gel and hairspray, and I came home to work on the research some more. Hours later, I found the answer. And when I called Jean to tell her, she couldn't believe it. Nonetheless, we were both very happy. After all, as much as I didn't want "pinwheel head", she certainly didn't want my sporting it as a walking advertisement!

Some of what I learned in that bout of research was well known. For example, when we are undergoing chemotherapy, we know that fast growing cells are destroyed. That's the concept behind chemotherapy: cancer cells multiply very rapidly; something that kills fast growing cells can keep the multiplication rate down and even reverse it if it can kill cells faster than they can reproduce. Scalp cells are fast growing cells, as are the cells in hair follicles. So while we lose our hair, we also slough off dead scalp cells. The problem arises when we quite naturally just wash our bare scalps with soap and rinse. After a while we begin to develop what I now call "chemo cap", that is a combination of soap and dead scalp cells that ultimately form plugs that close the pores on the scalp and keep the new hair trapped—ingrown, if you will—and we inevitably end up with less dense hair and another "age related problem".

So, when we are without hair, we need to do more than just wash our heads as we do the rest of our bodies. We need to exfoliate the scalp while it is hairless. Think of stylish men with nicely shaped heads who shave their heads every day because they like the look of it. With that shaving, they are also taking away dead skin cells which may have otherwise combined with soap residue to create a sort of scale on the scalp. That's what many of us get—chemo cap. So, we need to exfoliate our scalps while they are hairless and as the new hair begins to grow in after treatment! Then, when the hair is ready to grow back in, the pores on the scalp are open, and the follicles have room to sprout.

There are several ways to accomplish this exfoliation, but we have to be careful not to be too rough on the skin itself. Gentle exfoliation is the goal here. So, had I known then what I know now, I would have used a facial quality cleanser on my head, making sure that it was an exfoliating formula so it would remove those dead cells that combined with the soap film. You can make a gentle exfoliating scalp scrub by mixing a little brown sugar or sea salt into baby shampoo and using that on your head every day. The solution to my problem, so many years after my second challenge with hair recovery, is a product made by Paul Mitchell called Tea Tree Scalp Treatment. I'm not sure it isn't a bit strong for someone who is undergoing treatment, but after treatment, when the hair has started to grow in, it's amazing. It's refreshing and soothing as you work it through your hair and gently massage it over your scalp. The Tea Tree oil moisturizes the scalp, and it all shampoos out easily, product and dead cells alike. I still use Nioxin shampoo, and there are now four or five lines of products for different hair types to choose from, and the products you might want to try are readily available on line if the full selection is limited at your beauty supply store.

I found the Paul Mitchell exfoliating treatment at our local beauty supply store, and it is also available on line. The Nioxin products are a bit pricey, but worth it when you begin to get your hair back, and the Mitchell Tea Tree therapy is quite reasonable in price.

Whatever method you ultimately decide to use, exfoliating the scalp is crucial for long-term cancer survivors. I'm almost willing to bet that if women began to exfoliate their scalps when they became eligible for AARP membership, we might not have all the exposed scalps that we do.

In any case, for me, now that my hair volume is back to "near yellow dog" stage and still growing, I can again live Khalil Gibran's advice: "Forget not that the earth delights to feel your feet and the winds long to play with your hair." Mine is blonde again, and, like Hillary, I am amused!

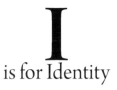

I

is for Identity

Ours is a family of readers. Books have been part of my life always. Our mother read to us (even when we were adults, in fact), and I learned to read for myself when I was three because my five years older sister loved to play "school". So, when she was eight and in third grade, learning to read on her own, she would come home, set me up at a little table and teach me what she had learned that day. As you can see, I've been listening to and reading stories for a long time.

One of the earliest stories I remember identifying with is "Little Red Riding Hood". My first connection to the story, I think, was the idea of going to visit Grandmother and taking her a basket of goodies. We lived with Mother's parents for a while, so that connection between child and grandparent that the story presented painted a clear picture for me of myself as the little girl going down the path to Grandmother's house. (The words to the Thanksgiving song, "Over the river and through the woods, to Grandmother's house we go" have the same effect).

I never gave much thought to the wolf, though, until I was five years old and had my tonsils removed. What a dirty trick that turned out to be! They told me I would just go to sleep for a while, and then when I woke up I would be able to eat all the ice cream I wanted. But--and here's where I understood that the wolf was not nice even if he did dress up like Grandma herself--nobody bothered to mention how sick I would be, and how sore my throat would be. Most wolf-like of all, though, was that not one single person, even my older siblings who had been through it before me, not one told me how awful ice cream tastes when it is flavored with ether!

Then two years later, just long enough to be lulled into a false sense of security about the actual dark capacities of wolves, I smashed my elbow in a mid-air crash with a much larger kid in a very competitive game of Kick the Can. After several attempts at trying to fix it, I was sent to a big hospital, where they put me under and inserted some wires in there to hold the bones together. And when I finally got out of that prison of a hospital, I had a year of physical therapy, which was really painful—especially for a little kid who now fully understood that the walk through the forest and meeting up with the wolf could end up very badly. After all, both Granny and Red were gobbled up by the wolf before that story ended! Why, if it hadn't been for the woodsman who happened to stop by and cut them out of the wolf's belly and then put an end to him, it would have instead been the end of Little Red and her grandmother.

Fairy tales are a door to both psychology and philosophy, and I think I've always been a philosopher, which has made more than one person a bit crazy, coming as it does with more questions than answers. I wondered where I went when they put me under the anesthetic—never mind how I felt when they called it "putting me to sleep" which I knew we had once had to do to a family dog. With the tonsils, I wondered whether or not I was the same person now that they had removed a part of me and with my elbow, I wondered if I was the same person now that they had put something into me.

In both cases, I decided I was the same person, but my body had been subjected to some unexpected experiences, not unlike Little Red when she was swallowed by that very scary wolf. And even though the woodsman, disguised as a series of doctors, had saved me, I was now officially scared. My body still worked for the most part, but it was forever changed, and I had a solid wariness about whether people would be wolves or woodsmen if I hurt myself again.

I was, as a child, developing a story about my Self, my body and the medical procedures that were being done to me, based on a fairy tale that made perfect sense under the circumstances. That story of mine, though certainly immature, was one of a person who was strong enough to go through very scary things and come out of them as a whole person, if not a whole body. I was a person who, though afraid of doctors—some of them total strangers—and other people in various styles of "wolves' clothing" could come through whatever they did to me-- changed, and yet the same.

Now, I could just as easily have developed a story that focused on nothing but the fear. I could have developed one that centered on the pain. I could have created one that made me out to be a victim. And I can't deny that even in my interpretation of the story, I carried around plenty of fear of "wolves" of every kind.

Fortunately, I was not done with Little Red Riding Hood. I say "fortunately" because I hadn't even begun to understand the story. In fact, I hadn't yet heard or read the real story! The one I knew had managed to make the woodsman the hero of the tale, and that wasn't quite true. There was, as the late commentator Paul Harvey used to say, "the rest of the story".

When I studied for my Master's Degree in 1989 and '90, I did a great deal of work with the ideas of the great depth psychologist, Carl Jung, and his notions of archetypes as represented in dreams, art and stories. I turned once again to "Little Red Riding Hood" and found a whole different version of the story!

In this version, Little Red goes through the woods, gets distracted from the path by the flowers, meets the wolf and spills the beans about going to Granny's house, finds a funny looking Grandma, gets swallowed up by that nasty old wolf and is then released from the belly of the wolf by the woodsman. No surprises there. But, in this version, Red doesn't stand by while the woodsman takes care of the big, bad wolf. Oh, no! Red essentially says to the woodsman "Stand back, sir!", and she begins to gather as many big stones as she can carry and puts them in the belly of the unconscious canine. Then she sits beside him and using the tools of Gran's sewing basket carefully closes up the wolf's belly with what I imagine are perfect little renditions of the blanket stitch, tidy and very sturdy.

Then all three humans (I see Red still on the floor while Grandma and the woodsman look on) wait patiently for the wicked wolf to waken. He sees the tall, strong woodsman standing over him, heavy axe in hand, and is frightened beyond fright, so he tries to run away. But first he has to try to stand up and, of course, with all those stones weighing him down, he has a desperate time of it! At the end of the story, Red and the others watch as the conquered old wolf, all the caginess gone from him now, work oh-so-very hard to drag himself back out into the forest, never again to do anyone any harm.

Can you imagine how Grandma and the woodsman both celebrated Little Red's heroic deed? Can you imagine how proud she was of herself for having thought of such a punishment and having the tools to make it happen? How clever, this girl! How creative is Red! How wise she is to use the tools of her femininity to battle the old dog! Of course she had the help of the woodsman—couldn't have done it without him. Of course she knew she had the support of her family--you can practically hear Granny cheering her on! But Red—the little girl in the red cape, skipping through the forest, stopping to investigate the flowers, seemingly not paying attention to business perhaps—won the day!

By that version of the story at that time of my life, my thinking about myself was transformed. The Little Red Riding Hood who had been with me my whole life now had a completely new dimension: Red as hero!

That's the story I use to identify my Self to myself as I have struggled and continue to struggle with all the aspects of cancer treatment and survival over these past ten years. That image of my Self is the one that urges me to find answers to questions that seemingly have none but that I know must not be dismissed as simply a matter of aging or hypochondria or fear. That story of my Self is the one that keeps me bound to my computer for hours doing the necessary research for this book. That story of my Self is the one that brings up the courage to question the members of my medical team and the so-called "common wisdom".

The heroic Little Red Riding Hood is brave enough to go into the unfamiliar and frightening world of the forest, curious enough to enjoy the flowers and meet the old wolf head-on, wise enough to be grateful for all the help and support she receives, smart enough to come up with new solutions to problems, and skilled enough to carry them out. The heroic Little Red Riding Hood is me.

So, who are you? What story are you living? And even more important, which version of the story do you carry in your head? If you find that you are interested in pursuing the psychological impact of the stories you are living, I recommend you do a little reading on the subject. The books that have helped me most (in this order) are Bruno Bettleheim's classic, "The Uses of Enchantment: The Meaning and Importance of Fairy Tales"; Jean Shinoda Bolen's "Goddesses in Everywoman: Powerful Archetypes in Women's Lives"; and "Awakening the Heroes Within: Twelve Archetypes to Help us Find Ourselves and Transform our World" by Carol Pearson.

Each of us is living a story, and we tell ourselves that story and modify it throughout our lives. So it's important to know who we are and whose ideas we are reflecting back to ourselves. As Anais Nin, the late writer, said: "We don't see things as they are; we see them as we are"

Our whole lives, but especially our experiences related to cancer and the therapy we've undergone in order to treat it, are all deeply influenced by the stories we tell ourselves. So we must ask ourselves if we will be naïve innocents like the early Red Riding Hood or heroes as she ultimately becomes. The wisdom of one my favorite philosophers, the French existentialist, Jean Paul Sartre, is well worth paying attention to here. He said, "…nothing foreign has decided what we feel, what we live, or what we are." You see, it's all us.

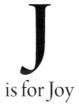

J

is for Joy

Long before cancer came into my life, I was quite confused about the nature of joy. I was like C. S. Lewis who said he wondered "whether all pleasures are not substitutes for joy". I certainly thought pleasure, gaiety, laughter, "good times", and fun were what joy was all about. .I thought "stuff"—a nice home, a car, a house, nice clothes, money—would bring happiness, which must be the same as joy. I thought getting attention from other people or praise for a job well done would make me joyful. I thought playing my social roles—daughter, wife, mother, homemaker, church goer, community participant—would lead to joy. It never once occurred to me to ask myself who I was or what I wanted for myself and for my life. And as a result of my lack of understanding, most of my younger years were lived in chaos.

Then life threw me a huge curve in the form of a divorce. I had failed in one of my most important roles! And that's when I began to live life in an almost constant state of chaos. I had to get a higher paying job, which introduced me to boredom for the first time ever. So I had to get an even higher paying job that would at least be interesting, but it involved a commute which took even more time away from my ability to fulfill my other roles. I had somehow decided I couldn't afford to keep my house, so I compensated for that lost role by using the extra money for newer, better clothes for my kids and me. A disastrous decision to re-marry followed, resulting in even more chaos and the need for an even higher paying job. That marriage might have worked if I had had a clue about myself and who I was and what I wanted and how to get it. But I didn't, so it didn't, and that meant another ill-defined choice to sell my house and find a higher paying job. This one came in management which took more of my time from my original designated social roles, and resulted in even more, even more hectic chaos.

I don't know if it was fortunate or unfortunate for me that a pretty high level of chaos was acceptable in the 1980s, at least in the crowd I joined. For me, it met some of those things I had always included in my definition of joy—praise, attention, money, "stuff". But now I know that I was always dissatisfied, that I created much of the chaos myself, I was physically compromised throughout all those years, not by illness but by conditions that almost always required some sort of surgery. And, of course, the medical issues simply added to the chaos and helped me in whatever part I played in creating it.

Let's face it: Chaos is exciting! In chaos we feel really alive! Remember what Hans Selye said about learning to live in a state of high adrenaline? Well, that state is a real WOW!, but it ultimately leads to a big fall because whatever you have that you think makes you feel happy, if not joyful, is built on sand. And when the collapse occurs, it is almost always total. It certainly was for me, and I had to start my life all over again. Oh, I tried to save what I had made, review it, revise it, find some way to hold onto it. But finally (finally is really a woman's word!) I realized I had to let all that go and begin again.

And so I went back to school. I had dropped out of college after high school in less than a semester because I had no plan—I certainly didn't want to be a *teacher*, a profession that had little support in my family—and I wanted to make some money, buy a car and find a husband. That's what I was supposed to do. Now, in my mid-forties I enrolled in our local community college, still no plan in mind, so I took the courses that I could fit between 9:00 am and 3:00 pm three days a week. Ultimately, that led to a two year degree in Liberal Arts, and because I had a credential in business management based on my experience, it also led to a part-time teaching position.

I loved college this time around! I remembered how much I had enjoyed high school, but then I liked extracurricular activities. This time I loved learning! I was awestruck by the things I learned every day. I realized that I wanted to do this. I had started it because I thought I could get another even higher paying job with a degree, but by the end of the first week, I knew I wanted to be in school for the rest of my life! For the first time, there was something on my personal agenda that I actually chose to do, that I actually wanted to do for me, and I didn't care (again for the first time) what anyone else thought about it. I wanted to KNOW! I had discovered the truth of Leonardo da Vinci's observation that "The noblest pleasure is the joy of understanding".

After I earned my Associate of Arts degree, I transferred to a fully accredited university with an alternate style educational plan. Designed for returning adults, the university offered a curriculum that met all the academic demands of a traditional university, but in every aspect of that curriculum, there was a focus on the interdisciplinary view and a second focus on consciousness, consciousness of self and the world in which self exists. Some Christians refer to themselves as being born again in the Lord. My first day on that campus I knew I had been reborn by the grace of God. I found home again on yet another college campus.

Consciousness studies opened the door to self-knowledge in a way that Plato himself would have approved. I learned the difference between my inner Self (essence/spirit) and my outer self (ego). While you might think that this emphasis on self-knowledge would build the ego, the experience was exactly the opposite. I had never felt so humble as I absorbed the wisdom of both the ages and modern advances from a multi-disciplinary view. I was so enthralled with my studies, that I decided I wanted a Master's Degree, and I got that, too. Then I wanted to teach Philosophy and Religious studies and Consciousness studies, all of which had exploded my world and shown me that those subjects involved practical skill sets that could be applied to the problems we all face in life in such a way as to make good decisions for our Selves instead of trying to appeal to the world around us. Those subjects make us part of the world around us and teach us how to make decisions that benefit the Self, which in turn always benefits the world around us. Life, I learned, is a circle, not a line, and it is in that circle that we find joy.

While my earlier life was painful, chaotic and clearly unsustainable (I say now), it was not wasted. I had learned, as Goethe said, "Only by joy and sorrow does a person know anything about themselves and their destiny. They learn what to do and what to avoid". I could not have learned what to do and what to avoid when I went to college at age 17. I had to have the sorrows involved in the messy life I created for myself, and I had to experience the false nature of the pleasures that I wrongly defined as joy before I could understand what Goethe was saying.

And then the real test of my newly recognized Self came in the form of aggressive, stage IIIB, systemic breast cancer. And two years later it came again in the form of ovarian cancer and in the style of a soccer ball. What in the heck do you do with that news? Well, as I've already said, when the breast cancer diagnosis was confirmed, I went to my mother's garden and watched her hummingbirds in action. After a few weeks, as we waited for the results of the CT scan that would tell us whether the cancer had metastasized, I went to the ocean and walked on the beach. Nothing brings joy to my Self faster and more completely than Mother Nature. As Albert Einstein wrote, "Joy in looking and comprehending is nature's most beautiful gift.", and in keeping with my multi-disciplinary approach to life, let me offer a relevant Native American Huron saying: "Listen to the voice of nature, for it holds treasures for us all".

But let me say here that cancer is a dreadful, scary disease, and its treatment is often just plain miserable. The surgery is painful, the chemo changes every aspect of your life, and radiation is exhausting-- don't let anyone tell you otherwise. And the second time is no better. Cancer treatment is not something you ever get used to. In fact, if anything, the more of it you have, the worse it gets. But there are still ways to keep your Self from dissolving into despair. I was first introduced to the work of the great mythologist, Joseph Campbell, when I went to community college, and was immersed in it when I transferred to the university. Campbell studied human beings through the lens of archetypes, or primary models. He said there are models in every society that demonstrate both human behavior and the ability we have to choose which of those behaviors we will decide to manifest in our lives, as well as the ability to choose to change them when they stop working for us. For cancer patients, I think these Campbell quotes are particularly helpful: "Find a place inside where there's joy, and the joy will burn out the pain" and "Participate joyfully in the sorrows of the world. We cannot cure the world of sorrows, but we can choose to live in joy".

So how can we participate joyfully in the sorrows of cancer treatment and long term cancer survival? How can we be joyful at the prospect that some of the toxic chemicals involved in stopping our cancer may have left permanent changes in our brains? How do we joyfully give up our expectations of a high quality life returning after our survival? Well, it's not easy, but there are ways.

The first way, of course, is nature. Daniel Boone was the younger brother of my great-, great-, great-, great, great-grandmother, and he said, "One day I undertook a tour through the country, and the diversity and beauties of nature I met within this charming season, expelled every gloomy and vexatious thought In such a diversity it was impossible I should be disposed to melancholy" A wise man, my ancestor.

Both times I had cancer I was in the midst of chemotherapy as early Spring rolled around. I experienced then, and still do now, absolute, clear, unabashed joy at the sight of the first daffodil each year. Imagine! That thing that looked like some kind of dried up, worthless chunk of onion or garlic that had been forgotten many months ago, could be put in the ground in October with a little bone meal, totally ignored throughout the winter, and then produce—sometimes surrounded by the remains of snow—a beautiful, bright yellow blossom! Who could have imagined that? Once again, to quote my Uncle Daniel, "Nature [is] a series of wonders, and a fund of delight".

We can keep a journal where we write down all of our frustrations, anxieties, sorrows and pain and lock it away, memorialized but not living. I always suggest that people who keep a journal end every entry with something that made them happy that day. It may be a day where you had to really look hard for that daffodil or its seasonal or human equivalent, but it's there some-where. Remember Goethe: you can choose.

We can bring beauty into our lives. One of the things my consciousness studies introduced me to is art. And when cancer became part of my life, so did a serious interest in art. I have original art, limited edition art and post-ers. I have impressionist works, as well as still lifes, watercolors, abstracts, and sketches. It doesn't matter what the piece is or if anyone else likes it or not. If it moves me, "speaks" to me, draws me in, then it's likely to end up on my wall. Schopenhauer, who was the most depressed and depressive philos-opher in all of Western philosophy to date, tells us that only saints can avoid the pain which constitutes all of life. BUT, even Schopenhauer says we mere mortals have a chance to experience joy in moments involving looking at art, listening to music, or being in nature. Very short moments, he says, but moments nonetheless! Khalil Gibran, the Sufi mystic, is much more posi-tive than Schopenhauer. He writes, "When you are joyous, look deep into your heart and you shall find it is only that which has given you sorrow that is giving you joy".

And we need not limit ourselves to looking at other people's art; we can make some ourselves. Oh, I know that whether we are artistic or not was pretty much decided for us when we were little children, but I'm going to tell you about art that anyone can do, and that will heal the Self of the artist. This art consists of drawing a circle (I use a dinner plate or a pie pan) on a piece of white paper with a lead pencil. Then the artist fills the circle with color. That's all. These circle drawings are called "mandalas", and the great depth analyst, Carl Jung, found that the Self responds in some very healthy way to these mandalas. He said there's something about the essence of our being that is moved by the sight of an empty circle. When I give this assignment to students, they always ask, "How do you want us to put in the colors?" Oh, boy, does that ever tell us that we don't do much to please ourselves! But after several times of hearing, "Just fill the circle with color and see what hap-pens", they get it, and they have fun. Besides being fun, there is something healing about mandalas. I've attended workshops with people who have suffered terrible tragedies, who have been healed by doing mandalas. They can be interpreted, if you're interested in that, but they don't have to be. But they must be respected. They should be hung up (masking tape works fine) so that you can look at them for awhile, and if you decide you're finished with one, you should make up a respectful ritual of some kind to destroy it because it is a part of your very soul trying to speak to you.

If you find you are interested in meditating with mandalas (a very good idea), I recommend "Meditating With Mandalas" by David Fontana (Dun-can Baird Publishers, ISBN: 1-844483-140-X). If you find you are interested in learning more about mandalas and how to interpret them, I recommend "Creating Mandalas: For Insight, Healing and Self-Expression" by Susanne F. Fincher (Shambhala, ISBN: 0-87773-646-4).

These mandalas are, as far as I'm concerned, little miracles at work, and for cancer patients and long term survivors, these words of Khalil Gibran have an important message for us: "Your pain is the breaking of the shell that encloses your understanding... And could you keep your heart in wonder at the daily miracles of your life, your pain would not seem less wondrous than your joy".

K
is for Kin

You can search far and wide in print and on the Internet, and you cannot find an ancient Greek god or goddess of the family. Now, I suspect that's at least partly because those Olympians were not very loving or kind or loyal. I mean, Cronus swallowed his male children at birth because it was told that he would be replaced by a son who walked the earth. If Rhea hadn't been wise enough with her final pregnancy to put the newborn Zeus in a hammock so his feet never hit the ground until he was big enough to put the old guy out of power, who can even imagine what might have happened to Western Civilization!

Zeus was unfaithful and had many progeny with both goddesses and humans, and he made no attempt to hide the fact that he had favorites among them. Hera, his wife, was a goddess of terrible unhappiness and wicked temper who treated her children horribly, even throwing her son, Hephaestus, off Olympus because he was born with a defect of his feet! And Zeus did awful things to his sisters and brothers and other members of his extended family.

Even without appropriate archetypal models, however, we can get a notion of how families and friends of long term cancer survivors are doing by looking once again at the research that is getting underway. We don't have a great deal of information, because, again, until recently there haven't been enough survivors to study the problem. Now, though, the research has begun, and we have some clues about what may be going on with the kin of long term cancer survivors, and we know absolutely that more work needs to be done to identify problems and find solutions in order to provide the support necessary for the survivor and the family perhaps for a lifetime.

In October of 2011, the Mayo Clinic published an article entitled, "Cancer Survivors: Reconnecting With Loved Ones After Treatment", in which they said by way of introduction, "Your friends and family love you and are worried about you—but they sometimes have strange ways of showing it... [and] one barrier to a smooth transition out of cancer treatment is the reaction [of] friends and family... [so] navigating relationships is a challenge for cancer survivors transitioning to life after treatment".

The Mayo authors identify several "common scenarios", which some of us have already experienced. When we were diagnosed, our families had to change quickly. Responsibilities changed, as did roles, and when projected results did not come into being, frustration was often the result.

In 2007 Mary E. Morris, BSN, MS; Marcia Grant, RN, DNSc, FAAN; and James C Lynch, PhD published an article entitled "Patient-reported family Distress Among Long-term cancer survivors" in which they compared five studies conducted by reputable institutions to begin to determine the quality of life of cancer patients who had survived for three to eight years from diagnosis. They found "Significant levels of patient-reported family distress to illness were reported in all five studies". The results of their findings were presented in the form of a quality of life model involving four major categories of well-being--physical, psychological, social and spiritual—as perceived by the survivor. Each of the four major categories had several subscales related to such things as strength/fatigue, anxiety/depression, family/finances/work, and meaning/religiosity respectively. The authors concluded that "only distress associated with diagnosis and treatment was identified as more stressful" than the distress experienced by families of long-term survivors.

Part of this distress comes from the fact, as published under "Survivorship" by the Emory University Winship Cancer Institute, that "having cancer may change the way that a patient relates with friends and colleagues". They also point out ways in which friends and family may respond to the cancer patients, saying "While some relationships provide needed support, other relationships may unexpectedly lead to frustration... Many want to offer support, but they just do not know how... [and then] After treatment ends, some friends, family, or co-workers may tend to show less support due to their belief that the cancer is gone [and the patient is back to normal].

The fact is, however, that many of us may never be the same as we were before cancer. We are, for the most part, permanently changed in a variety of ways, and it doesn't appear that there is a particular model for how we've changed, so not only are there no archetypal models to follow, there are no models at all. We are left to find our own way, each of us, as best we can. It can be said that we now suffer from a chronic condition that doesn't really have a specific name of its own, but it affects us similarly. We are often forgetful, confused, disorganized, sweaty, exhausted, in pain, and anxious or depressed, and we hate it. We do our best to hide it, but our families are hard to fool, and so we have to address it because as Michael J. Fox, a chronic illness survivor whose fame and wealth give him no protection, says, " Family is not an important thing, it's everything".

The beginning of the family is, of course, the couple who first established it. And an essential ingredient of the successful family is a successful relationship between the two of them, which without a doubt includes sexuality. For that, we do have an archetype from ancient Olympus, the beautiful, passionate, sensuous Aphrodite, the original sex kitten. She is married to the very homely and disabled, but fabulously gifted and artistic Hephaestus, but she is madly and passionately in love with the war god, Aries—beauty and caring in the first relationship and love and war in the second!

All too often the long term cancer survivor couple have lost their passion or are afraid to try to express it. They remember how it used to be, the way my favorite poet, Marge Piercy, described is in her poem "Raisin pumpernickel"

> The tomcat is a ready lover. He can do it at dawn
> when the birds are still yawning, he can do it
> while the houseguest walks up the drive, do it after
> four parties and an all-night dance, on a convenient floor.
>
> So are you able.

The tomcat, of course, must also have a willing and able partner, but it may be troublesome for couples to resurrect those feelings after that terrible disease, which may already have made them work through anxieties about body image, possible pain, and performance. Now there is a new set of problems, and each may be thinking as (again) Marge Piercy writes in her poem "A penetrating cold",

> my emptiness curls around itself wishing
> to sleep through the winter of your absence.

And neither may know that there is relief to be had and life to be reclaimed. They may be anxious about discussing it with each other, much less their physicians. Those who suffer this loss of intimacy know only that nothing has been the same since their lives were consumed by the evil portrayed in Marge Piercy's poem, "The bottom line":

> That white withered angel cancer
> steals into a house through cracks,
> lurks in the foundation, the walls…
> We come to mistrust the body
> a slave to be starved to submission
> an other that can like a rabid dog
> turn on and bite a separate me.

The answer lies, I think, in understanding and managing the long term after effects of chemotherapy. It's found in understanding that the survivor's memory and emotions and sheer competencies have been permanently altered. Once that is understood, all the rest depends on kindness, understanding and patience.

Those are easy words to write, but not easy words to live. So let me add another: affection. We are not much taught in our culture how to express affection. As the early 20th century American journalist, Agnes Smedley, wrote, "Like all my family and class, I considered it a sign of weakness to show affection; to have been caught kissing my mother would have been a disgrace, and to have shown affection for my father would have been a disaster". But, if sex is not available at a given time, holding hands is, hugging is, cuddling is, dancing is, talking is. We place so much emphasis on sexuality in our culture that we sometimes come to think that's all there is to an intimate relationship, but that is so untrue. Lust has little to offer in the long term without affection. With affection (and the understanding and attention it presumes to contain) lust, desire, and sexual expression will return. And if it doesn't, although there is no reason to support the idea that cancer survivors and their partners are at any greater risk for separation than any other couples, the intimate practices that develop from intentional expressions of affection will be enough. The National Cancer Institute reports in its "Facing Forward: Life After Cancer Treatment" that about half of women and more than half of men who have had treatment for cancer of the breast or reproductive organs report long-term sexual problems. So these things may be here to stay, and if they are, you must rely on what is available to you: attention and affection. As George Bernard Shaw once wrote, "If you cannot get rid of the family skeleton, you may as well make it dance". Or, even better, you can concentrate on another goddess who is not well known as Aphrodite. She is, however, much more important to the long term cancer surviving couple. She is the goddess Philotes, who is the goddess of friendship **but even more importantly** the goddess of affection and sexual intercourse!

The adult couple in the family are, of course, not the only ones who are affected by the long term after effects of chemotherapy. The entire family is. So what can be done to ease the tension with children? A teenager can understand that the tension in the family stems from the after effects of chemotherapy. That undoubtedly will be extremely frustrating for any child who has been through the same fears and stresses of cancer treatment and expected all to be well once the parent was deemed to be cancer free. Everything should go back to normal—that's what we all think. And when they don't, it's as difficult for the teenager whose freedom to grow and explore the world may already have been stifled by the parent's disease. The response from the teenager is very likely to be anger and resentment. Once again, frequent applications of affection are the answer. Open communication about how frustrating all this is for everyone, allowing the teen to return to "normal" to the greatest extent possible, and being kind and asking for kindness in return is the answer. Just remember, the most important part of good open communication is **listening!**

Small children need exactly what they needed during the cancer treatment. They need to feel secure. And the same people can provide that sense of security when the cancer survivor can't. The other parent, older siblings, Grandparents—all can help the child.

And we must learn to manage these long-term effects because they involve so much loss of self and frustration. But think about this. Those of us who are long-term survivors have had the cancer and the treatments, including chemotherapy and radiation and surgery, and we are now cancer free. Some of us have been cancer free and out of treatment for five or even ten years. How can we possibly blame our disorderly, forgetful, mindless behavior on cancer or our treatment? Why would we even think to do so? Well, we can blame it, for all the good it will do. It is enough to know that it is real, and knowing that it is a part of our reality, we can deal with it. We have total control over this part of it! We had no control over the first part. So we can choose how we deal with how we feel.

Hestia (Vesta in the Roman pantheon) was a virgin goddess, so we can't really think of her as a goddess of the family. But one of the things Hestia is responsible for is the spiritual aspects of the home. In every ancient Greek home the eldest daughter was responsible for the utensils involved in worshipping the special god or goddess of that home and family. The eldest male in the household conducted the ritual(s), but the physical objects used in the ritual(s) were taken care of by the eldest daughter. Then, when the eldest daughter married, she would gather together a sort of spiritual "hope chest" containing the tools for rituals which she would take into her own home and take care of the spiritual needs of her family by taking care of the very tools through which that spirit was expressed.

That basic spiritual expression of the family in the home is something we survivors (or our eldest daughters) can be responsible for as a new contribution to a family that has been through much and can but look forward to more. There is so much to be grateful for. Even the body that sometimes is so impossible to manage is the one that got you through phase one in pretty good condition overall. It's true that we are not perfect, but then, we never were nor ever will be. So we should sing. We should find ways to express our frustration and anger without dumping them on the people we love. Some say home is the one place where you can let yourself go and be as completely miserable as you want, and no one can judge you. Oh, I disagree with that. Home should be a sanctuary for every member of the family. Home should be a place of warmth and kindness and, most of all, affection, even (and maybe especially) for ourselves.

If we choose it to be so, there is nothing ahead for patients and their kin but hope. Remember Pandora of our ancient Greek stories. Pandora was the first woman, and her name means "all-gifted" because when she was created, all the gods gave her unique and sensuous gifts. Then her curiosity got the best of her, and she opened a jar (or box) that contained all the evils of mankind, except one. When Pandora opened the box and let loose all the world's troubles, the one thing left was hope. I think part of hope, the thing that supports hope perhaps more than any other, besides affection, is humor, and so we can use the wisdom of the actor, Ralph Fiennes, "One of the things that binds us as a family is a shared sense of humor". We can all work on developing that.

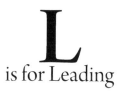

L
is for Leading

Those of us who are long term survivors of cancer treatment have become, like it or not, leaders. We are on the leading edge of all the research that's being done to determine what sort of nervous system damage the A-C chemotherapy cocktail may have caused. Because these after effects occur even years after treatment, we are leading in the most basic research through the Internet and our various support groups in determining that they are *real!* We are the leaders in reporting the after effects to our oncologists or primary care doctors, which, in turn, has resulted in the beginning of research to determine their cause. And we lead when we acknowledge these after effects and take action to manage them as best we can. But we must now take our leadership more public. We must make people, from our families to our physicians to our fellow survivors, aware that having had cancer and having been treated with chemotherapy consisting of Adriamycin, Cytoxan and the other elements of that cocktail, we are not done with cancer. As much as we wish we were not only surviving, but healthy and the same as we were before that first diagnosis, we aren't. We have to lead people into an understanding that we are not just whining, and that we would "GET OVER IT" if only we could.

I understand that the idea of being a leader in anything is a foreign one to many of us. The information contained in this book will help you, and those who hear you will become more patient about the behaviors we survivors exhibit as a result of our having survived cancer treatment. If we look at the story of the warrior goddess, Athena, from Greek mythology, she can help teach us how to go about being a leader. Here's the story:

Zeus, the chief god of the ancient Greek pantheon, had amazing abilities. One of them was the ability to have a child by himself. He carried these motherless children in his thigh or, in the case of Athena, in his head. One day Zeus had a terrible headache—the worst headache imaginable. Ancient Greece had no ibuprofen, of course, and the headache became so unbearable that he called upon his son, Hephaestus, who was an iron worker, and ordered him to do something about the god's headache. Hephaestus was not a favored child, so we can't be sure of his motivation, but he took up an axe and smashed the blade into his father's forehead. Well, the most amazing thing happened. A full grown, fully armored woman sprang out of Zeus's head! He named her Athena, and the City of Athens is named for her. Athena became the most favored child of Zeus, so much so that he put her in charge of war and even told her, and never anyone else, where he kept the thunderbolt which was the Zeusian prototype of a nuclear weapon.

Now, the interesting thing about Athena for we who are long term survivors of cancer and cancer treatment is that although she was the goddess of war and had full access to the thunderbolt, she never became angry and never used any tool of war. Instead, she planned with the armies. She advised the heroic warriors described in Homer's mythology. She saved the men who failed to follow her advice and got themselves into trouble such as Achilles and Odysseus. She was a brilliant tactician and a goddess of grace and peace. She led the armies by teaching them and helping them heal when they were undone.

Athena is a perfect model for everyone who learns about the long term after effects of chemotherapy and other cancer treatment. The things we're talking about in this book are anything but widely known. As I mentioned in the Doctors chapter, even our physicians don't know what is being learned in laboratories around the world. The research is too new and involves too great a variety of disciplines for them to keep up. So, it's up to us!

I feel the same as the television actress and reporter, Karen Duffy, who suffers from a terrible incurable disease, when she said, "I never expected in a million years that I would have the honor to become an advocate of women's health care and education, and I'd dive on a live grenade to get this message out..." That's how I feel about this book and the information in it, and I hope all my readers will join me in an Athena-like leadership role, and spread this word to everyone and in every way that we can. Peter Drucker, a famous management consultant, commented that "Management is doing things right; leadership is doing the right things." Taking a leadership role in the effort to help make patients and health care providers aware of the problems faced by an unknown, but very large number of cancer patients and what is being done about them is the right thing to do.

So you might well ask: "How do we go about that?" And my answer is, begin with your primary care physician and your oncologist. If you aren't comfortable talking about the heavier scientific components of the problem, give them a copy of this book. The reference list is full of authoritative sources they can consult.

Take this message to your local cancer support group, and if you belong to an online support group, take it there as well. As the late Norman Cousins said in his book, "Anatomy of an Illness", the story of how he cured himself of a very serious disease, "If something comes to life in others because of you, then you have made an approach to immortality." Now that may seem a bit excessive, but it isn't really, because the people you teach and lead will lead and teach others, and as this disease strikes younger and younger people, the information you're spreading crosses generations, and you have no idea where your words will go.

I know almost everyone is afraid of public speaking. I know that because any number of surveys taken over the years show that the fear of death is second on the list of people's fears. First on the list is public speaking. But if you do what I'm asking you to do, you won't really be doing public speaking at all. You'll be passing along extremely important information to people whom you know, either personally or by way of the Internet. That's all. There's nothing to be afraid of in that. Besides, the writer, Seth Grodin tells us that "Being a leader gives you charisma …", so this task of helping your medical team and your fellow patients and survivors just might take you to places you never thought you'd see.

When you help lead the dissemination of this information, you cannot know how much help and support you provide. Quoting Norman Cousins again: "The human body experiences a powerful gravitational pull in the direction of hope. That is why the patient's hopes are the physician's secret weapon. They are the hidden ingredients in any prescription." I think helping to bring people hope is the most important thing we can do to honor our own struggles in this never-ending journey with cancer. For me, it gives real meaning to the whole terrible experience. I hope that works for you, as well.

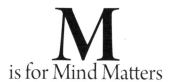

M
is for Mind Matters

I had a really terrific opening line for this chapter, and a little story to go along with it, but I forgot it!

No, not really. The story I have for you is the story of the goddess, Mnemosyne, who was the Ancient Greek goddess of memory. She was a very powerful goddess because memory is the gift that makes humans different from all the other creatures of the earth. She was the mother of the Muses, the goddesses of music, art, poetry and the sciences, and she gives us memory so that we can, as the website, Goddess Gift tells us, "reason, predict and anticipate outcomes [which] is the very foundation for civilization". Without memory and the ability to reason, we would not have the talents governed by the Muses. And in ancient times, memory was critical to the continuation of civilization because there were no books, and oral histories or stories were the only means of educating new generations.

With memory being such a basic element of human existence, it is no wonder that those of us who have survived systemic chemotherapy and begin to forget things, worry. A lot! But one thing we don't have to worry about is Alzheimer's disease, because people who suffer from Alzheimer's lose their memories. We do not lose our memories, but we may well have a very difficult time accessing them—from remembering a person's name to forgetting how to do an ordinary task. I often have an experience in class where I forget a student's name when I'm trying to answer a question, and then I'll find I don't remember the answer either. But in about half an hour or so, as I'm on my way home from the college, I'll remember both with absolute clarity. Fatigue (or the lack of energy) is the most common complaint of long term cancer survivors, and, unfortunately, it makes every other symptom worse.

Names are a very interesting part of these post chemo effects, and not just because we forget the names of people we've known for a long time. I've recently developed a new trick where I just rename the people—without their permission and (hopefully) without their knowing it. But sometimes you help them find out! I have a student whose name is Kenny. Kenny has been a student of mine for over a year. I know Kenny's name as well as I know my own, but one day I began calling him Randy. Sadly, he was doing a presentation that day, so I used his "new" name a lot, and everyone in the class knew I was off the mark. I apologized to Kenny for that one.

But the newest one is something I can't apologize for because I can't let the person involved know I've renamed her. We have a new staff person this year whose name is Susan. She works in our library, so I have had a great deal of contact with her in the process of doing research for this book. Somehow, somewhere absolutely unknown to me, I decided her name is Heidi. Now I know very well her name is not Heidi, so I work very, very hard to get the name Susan in my mind AND on a note before I meet with her or speak with her on the telephone. What else can I do? Well, I do laugh at myself every time I think "I have to go see Heidi"!

I don't recall ever forgetting my own name, but just to make sure I don't make a complete fool of myself in that regard, I always write it on the board in my college classroom so people can read it when they come in, and if my mind has left for the grocery store while my body stays at the college, I at least have a reminder!

The worst, though, as a college professor, is when I am lecturing on a specific philosophy or philosopher, and the name, which I spoke confidently only moments before, is gone. I don't usually use notes when I lecture, so I often find myself literally at a loss for words. I'm very open with my students about having had cancer and about my chemo brain problems, so I look for a "helper student" early on in the semester. Then when I draw a blank, I just stop and say, "Okay. Where was I?" And my helper students get me back on track. If I've put a good bit of information in whiteboard notes, I'll ask the helper to take them down verbatim and then let me copy them after class so that I'll have them, too. When I forget the rest of "In the 5th century BCE, Plato wrote in 'Republic' that ....", all I can do is ask them where I was going, and then we trace back until I find a train of thought that sounds familiar so I can start again. The plan that works best for me is being honest and then trying to make fun out of it all. I can only hope at least some of the students share my sense of humor!

I am fortunate to work in the field of education. That means my brain is being used at pretty high levels for some part of every day. Since I use a relaxed, inter-active teaching style, I have to be on my toes whenever I'm with students, because I never know what they are going to ask or what opinions they're going to offer or what they're going to begin to argue with me about. I have to be able to pull up an answer or help them explore the opinion or offer up a counter argument at any moment. Sometimes I give an incomplete or incorrect answer to a question, and then I have to be sure to remember to correct myself at the next class meeting.

I'm learning to write things down in a planner—it's really slow learning process for me because I'm still not used to not being able to remember all the details of my life. Now I have to learn to remember to look at the planner!

I use sticky notes all the time, but there is some disagreement about whether or not that's a good idea. I've used them ever since they were invented, and I love them. Some people say, though, that we don't need lots of little pieces of paper floating around with reminders on them. I do have a program of sticky notes on my computer, and that's working pretty well because the reminder is always right in front of me. I find I need to take care of the things I put on my desktop pretty quickly, though, because if I don't, they tend to just become part of the scenery.

I have been using my own method of managing the "to do" list that I described in "Energy" for a long time. I find now I have to be even tougher with myself and not give myself more than I can comfortably handle. The motivating element in that process is knowing that if I do too much today, then I'll likely be able to do nothing tomorrow, so I'm not just trying to keep my stress down, I'm really trying to manage my "bars" in advance. It's not easy, but I get better at it all the time. For example, I used to set aside a full day to do nothing but grade papers. Now I set aside a few hours over two or three days to do the same job. Because my brain is really a tool of my trade, I have to help it in every way that I can.

Writing this book has been an incredible exercise for my brain because the research took me into areas I knew absolutely nothing about. So it's been a constant process of researching, learning what the research is telling me by researching some more or asking questions of experts, and then translating that information for my readers so they will be able to make sense of it and speak about it comfortably.

I really wanted this book to be entertaining as well is informative and even groundbreaking. So developing the angles I wanted to take to present the information was an ongoing mental exercise, as was finding the ancient Greek models—many of which I'd never heard of before, or I'd heard of them but didn't know their stories—was both informative and fun. I'll be using them in future classes.

I'm not sure what I'll do now that the book is done, but now that I know how important it is to keep thinking, I'll find something. But this is going to be a tough act to follow! One thing I know for sure now, though, is that once we become aware of the need to consciously USE our brains as opposed to spending them on worry, almost everything can be a mental exercise. We just take our brains for granted and don't even think about what wondrous things they are. But it seems to me that my brain appreciates the attention I'm giving it. It deserves at least as much attention as my hair!

Dealing with people in normal circumstances if you have a blank moment and try to explain it, you'll hear "Oh, I have that all the time", and I just want to scream. I think that's one of the most difficult things about the cognitive impairment portion of this problem: You simply cannot describe it adequately. Everyone misplaces their keys; everyone walks into a room and forgets why they're there; everyone forgets someone's name; everyone gets confused; everyone gets frustrated and sometimes expresses that frustration through anger. But what we have is different. The physical aspects of chemo brain—changes in vision, hearing, smell and taste, balance—are harder to counter with an assurance of shared experience, but, of course, they can be dismissed with the catchall "we're all getting older". But the intellectual-emotional components are almost impossible to convey to anyone other than another long-term survivor!

I find there's no point in trying to explain what this is to any "normal" person because they'll say they have it, too; or they'll tell me I should get on with my life and forget about cancer; they'll say that I seem to be completely normal to them. On that last one I've come to the conclusion that either they are not very observant, or I'm doing a great job of playing the role of my pre-treatment self. Either way, I win!

As I've said, when I found Dr. Deitrich's 2006 article, I danced even though he was suggesting that I had brain damage from chemo. A thing with a name (or several names) that is acknowledged and being studied is ever so much better than a thing everyone thinks I'm imagining!

And we must all remember to hold on to hope because a central nervous system problem that causes a type of brain injury, although a bit scary, will ultimately lead to a myriad of answers. We will learn which drugs or combinations of drugs are most dangerous and perhaps deliver them differently or reduce dosages. We'll find out if some people are more prone to developing cognitive problems than others. We'll find other drugs or combinations of drugs that are less toxic. In other words, knowing that there is a problem, and having a very clear basic understanding of what the symptoms can be and which neurotoxic cancer treatments are most dangerous and how that dangerous mechanism works in the central nervous system and brain, we will find answers.

We already are learning how to diagnosis the problems through neurological testing of various kinds. In some treatment centers associated with university medical centers, neurologists are being included prior to the beginning of treatment so baseline MRIs can be obtained and considered in designing the treatment protocol.

We live at a good time; a time of great discovery and we are the Galileos of our time. A year ago I was completely frustrated by what was happening to me and the fact that Dr. Pirruccello and I could not find the answers. Then last summer, the University of Rochester/Harvard University team made me dance, and I've been dancing ever since. And when a problem arises or confusion with another person evolves, I just say to myself: "Self, it's just the chemo stuff", and I carry on. The only thing that can sit me down hard now is my darn cell phone like body, but I've learned that I just have to let it have its way. Fighting that only makes everything much, much worse.

N

is for Nervous System

As I've made my way inevitably to this very important chapter, I've often thought I would have to put on my entire ensemble of academic regalia (the fancy term used by the people who sell caps and gowns) to tell you about the scientific breakthrough announced on June 11, 2011 at the meeting of the Oncology Society. I mean this involves some really *intimidating* scientific words, some of which I'm still trying to learn to pronounce. And then I realized I didn't have to do that; there was another way. I'd have to write those words once, but then I could give them new names. So, let's continue with our tale.

"A TALE OF KINGS AND KNIGHTS AND DAMSELS IN DISTRESS"

Part Three

After a time of celebration of the breakthrough the royal scientists and physicians had made that helped the knights and dames and damsels understand what was happening to them after being treated for cancer, and after the news had been carried to every nation, even those that had not engaged in the earlier wars, the kings began to wonder about this breakthrough. What was it exactly, they said. How did it all work, they asked. What will they do with it, they mused. So they called all the royal physicians and scientists from all their kingdoms and brought them together for a conference on the details of the breakthrough.

Well, those who had worked on the breakthrough over the years, and those who had succeeded in actually making it in the 11th year of the 21st century were both excited at the prospect of meeting and talking with each other as well as the royal heads of state. And at the same time, they were concerned that what they had discovered might once again put anxiety in the hearts of the dames and damsels and their knights. So it was with conflicted feelings that the royal scientists and physicians responded to the commands of their monarchs.

The royal physicians suggested that the royal scientists prepare and present their findings since the royal physicians were not all yet clear themselves about what the breakthrough meant. And so it was that the royal scientists from every kingdom from all around the world came to the center of the world to present their findings.

All the scientists from all the kingdoms presented the findings of their teams in the last five years. One team from Japan had studied the brains of women who suffered from and been treated for breast cancer, and they discovered that there was a reduction in the white matter in these women's brains.

The kings were confused because they had always heard about grey matter, and how important grey matter was in developing intelligent, high information people, which is what they wanted for their kingdoms. So the scientists explained to the monarchs that white matter is a massive collection of stem cells (beginner cells), progenitor cells (baby cells with lots of potential), glial cells (the manufacturers) that made a product called myelin which needed to be wrapped around the baby cells so they could develop their potential, and oligodendrocytes (wrappers) the cells that wrapped the myelin around the axons (tails) of the baby cells so that they could connect to the strings of similar cells that served the specific need that would allow the baby cells to manifest their potential.

In the central nervous system process, the royal scientists explained, the baby cells when properly wrapped would become neurons and would connect to other neurons to keep every aspect of the bodies of the people working properly. The neurons, they explained, were in the grey matter with which they were familiar. But it was in the white matter that the whole process began.

The kings and all the members of the court and all the knights and dames and damsels knew from articles in the media and information on the internet that their bodies shed dead cells all the time, and they knew that somehow the body, in its wisdom, replaced those cells most of the time. Those who had been in the war on cancer knew about cells because they talked about them all the time in their treatment. But they had thought the chemotherapy they endured would only kill cancer cells, hair cells and sometimes white blood cells.

The royal scientists explained that they had always thought that because of the membrane known as the blood brain barrier, the toxic chemotherapy cells being infused into the bloodstreams of patients would not be able to get through to any part of the brain. But, they said, this reduction in the amount of white matter indicated that cells were being affected by something.

They said that they had tested brain tissue in the laboratories and found little evidence of chemotherapeutic agents in the neurons. They explained that they did not know how the toxic agents would make their way into the brain, but they were confident that they had. Then, they explained, they could conclude that the toxic agents were in the brain because they found measurable levels of those toxins in the spinal fluid, which was the essence of the central nervous system.

Finally, they said, they began to wonder, as scientists are prone to do, if the damage was being done at the earliest stages of cell building—in the white matter.

The scientists explained that they knew that a baby cell consisted of a body with an axon, a sort of tail. They knew, they said, that the axon of each baby cell had to be wrapped with myelin, just like an electrical cord has to be wrapped in insulation. Like an electrical cord, when baby cells finally become neurons, they transmit electrical charges that operate the body just as electrical cords operate appliances. This insulation (myelin) they knew had to be wrapped to very specific standards, just as an electrical cord would be, so that the electrical charges could not break loose and cause a short circuit.

When the conference members reconvened, the monarchs, somewhat refreshed, indicated to the royal scientists that they could continue. Many of the people who were attending the conference who had been treated during the war on cancer were becoming a bit anxious with all this talk about something perhaps having happened to their brains because they only had a little information, and they had expressed their concerns to their friends and not the royal physicians.

Even so, the royal scientists moved ahead in their presentation, and what they had to say disturbed some of the people even more. They reminded the courts that the wrapper cells (oliogondendrocytes) had to do their jobs of wrapping the axons of the baby cells absolutely perfectly so that the insulation would be strong enough to prevent any short circuits.

What they had discovered, the royal scientists said, was that sometimes the wrapper cells were damaged by the toxic agents in the chemotherapy that fought cancer and often saved lives. They said that because the wrapper cells were damaged, they were not able to perfectly wrap the axons on the baby cells. Thus, as everyone could see, it was possible that some baby cells would not be properly or completely wrapped when they joined the units to which they were assigned to manifest their potential.

The crowd made a strange sound as all the people gasped in fear at this news. But the scientists bravely continued.

If, they said, a wrapper cell died from the toxic agents in the chemotherapy, then the baby cell might not get wrapped, and it might not be able to join its assigned family in order to fulfill its potential. That could leave a break in the chain of that particular function, and the person who had that break in his or her circuitry could have trouble completing the task controlled by that chain.

If, they said, a wrapper cell was damaged by the toxins, it might well be able to take the myelin from the producer cell and wrap the axon to the best of its ability, but not quite to specifications. In that case, they said, the baby cell might take its place in the chain of neurons with an innate weakness, and that weakness might cause a short circuit in that chain at any time—even five or ten years or more after the axon was wrapped.

The scientists explained that these short circuits, whenever they occurred, whether at the beginning of the wrapper's exposure to the toxic agents or at some later date when a weakness in the wrapping became apparent, could, indeed, be the reason why the people who had been treated with chemotherapy during the war on cancer would sometimes develop problems. The problems were many and varied. They could be with their memories, their ability to organize and complete tasks, their energy levels, their experience of pain, in their vision, hearing or taste sensations, in their sense of heat and cold, in their sleep patterns, and many other things that the scientists had not yet encountered.

You can imagine how the people felt, especially the dames and damsels and their knights. They had just been told they might have brain damage as a result of having survived their respective cancers!

But the royal scientists weren't finished. When the crowd had settled down again, they proceeded with their presentation. 'This is just the beginning', they said. 'We have known about this chemo brain after effect for many years, and now that we are on the trail of the cause, we have something to work with', they said. 'There are other conditions that involve myelination, and we can study them and learn from them', they said. 'There are many other types of brain injuries that result in the same sorts of symptoms our patients have', they said, 'and we can learn from them'. They said, 'What you have now is a condition with a name. What you have is now accepted as real. With reality and a name, you have hope', they said. 'And trust us', they said.

'We will not stop our work until we have answers for you and all the courageous survivors of the war on cancer and all the courageous people who face it in the future have a better way.'

The silence in the room was so profound, you could hear the proverbial pin drop. The scientists and physicians of the various courts began to be a bit anxious themselves as they wondered how the people would respond to their news. And then a roar went up from the crowd—a roar of approval, a roar of support.

No one in the crowd was under the false impression that a cure had been found. All of them knew there was much more work to do. But at the same time, they were, as the scientists had hoped, relieved to know that they weren't worse off, that they weren't losing their minds. And when the conference ended, with so many now high information people, the kings and all their courts rejoiced, not just over the breakthrough as they had before, but over what the breakthrough promised, not only for the future but for the long term survivors of the day.

"THE BEGINNING"

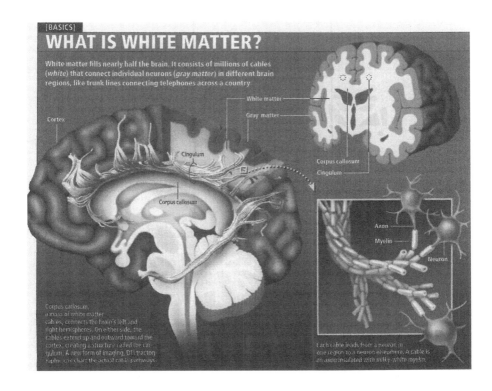

[BASICS]

WHAT IS WHITE MATTER?

White matter fills nearly half the brain. It consists of millions of cables (*white*) that connect individual neurons (*gray matter*) in different brain regions, like trunk lines connecting telephones across a country.

Cortex

White matter

Gray matter

Cingulum

Corpus callosum

Cingulum

Corpus callosum

Axon

Myelin

Neuron

Corpus callosum, a mass of white matter cables, connects the brain's left and right hemispheres. On either side, the cables extend up and outward toward the cortex, creating a structure called the cingulum. A new form of imaging, DTI tractography, can chart the actual cable pathways.

Each cable leads from a neuron in one region to a neuron elsewhere. A cable is an axon insulated with milky-white myelin.

WHAT IS WHITE MATTER

Scientific American, March, 2008

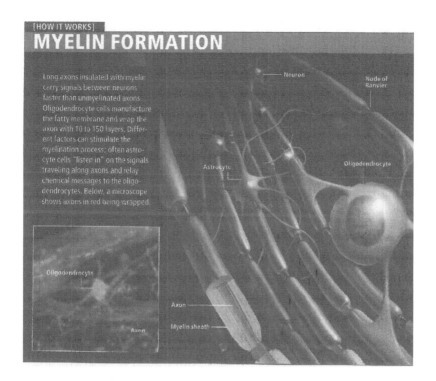

[HOW IT WORKS]

MYELIN FORMATION

Long axons insulated with myelin carry signals between neurons faster than unmyelinated axons. Oligodendrocyte cells manufacture the fatty membrane and wrap the axon with 10 to 150 layers. Different factors can stimulate the myelination process; often astrocyte cells "listen in" on the signals traveling along axons and relay chemical messages to the oligodendrocytes. Below, a microscope shows axons in red being wrapped.

Neuron

Node of Ranvier

Astrocyte

Oligodendrocyte

Oligodendrocyte

Axon

Axon

Myelin sheath

WHITE MATTER FORMATION

Scientific American, March, 2008

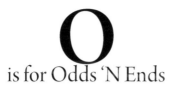

O
is for Odds 'N Ends

- ❖ Our cancer was problematic for other people, and so is our survival.

- ❖ The difficulties we experience with other people are different from those we face with family.

- ❖ Awareness of long term after effects of cancer treatment was first found in children.

- ❖ Hair loss is not the most traumatic part of having and being treated for cancer.

- ❖ Many cancer survivors do not return to work or return with fewer hours.

- ❖ It's unknown whether reduction in work is due to further illness or a priorities change.

- ❖ Employers cannot discriminate against cancer survivors.

- ❖ Socrates said "The unexamined life is not worth living", so examine yours.

- ❖ A code of ethics helps make life more meaningful.

- ❖ Chemotherapy survivors keep their memories but have trouble retrieving them.

- ❖ Alzheimer's patients lose their memories.

- ❖ Chemo fog results in nearly $300 million a year in direct costs and $250 million in indirect costs.

- ❖ Heat intolerance is much worse than menopausal hot flashes; many long-term survivors agree that chemo "broke their thermostats"—it did mine.

❖ Women who have been diagnosed with breast cancer often develop post traumatic stress disorder because of the possibility that the disease might be fatal.

❖ We used to frame our lives in terms of the births of our children, but now we tend to frame them in terms of before and after cancer.

❖ We have to do a better job of educating and finding support for spouses/partners.

❖ I worry every day about women with chemo after-effects being diagnosed as clinically depressed, medicated and sent on their way.

❖ We can both love God and be furious with God at precisely the same time, and it's okay.

❖ Never forget that if you got through all this stuff, you're one tough cookie!

❖ With all the political talk about changing Medicare or reducing programs for sick and disabled folks, not to mention a reluctance to provide care/insurance for everyone or to assure coverage for pre-existing conditions and no limit to treatment, we should all be paying close attention to what's going on in our state legislatures as well as Congress!

❖ Jamie S. Myers, an oncology nurse who contributed to Chemo Fog (see references) came up with a great name for this condition: CRCI for chemotherapy-related cognitive impairment. Cool!

❖ The changes in our cognition are mostly subtle, but that doesn't mean they aren't significant and can be ignored.

❖ Everyone agrees we don't know much about this CRCI, but almost everyone agrees it's real.

❖ There are records of patients reporting post-chemo cognitive impairment as far back as the late 1980's.

❖ Don't let anyone confuse neurotoxic with neurotic, ever!

❖ Sometimes the changes resulting from CRCI are very clear such as deafness. The actress, Kathy Bates can attest to that.

- In Chapter 19 of Chemo Fog the authors tell of a 1980 report by Dr. Peter Siberfarb, et al, which said they were surprised that some patients developed cognitive impairment due to the fact that the drugs given some patients "are known to not cross the blood brain barrier (BBB). And that's where we were (and many still are) until 2006.

- My friend who is fighting pancreatic cancer had a bad week.

- She has so much more pain than I did; I hate her cancer more than my own.

- I dripped all the way through classes today. New students must wonder what's wrong with me. I suppose I'll have to tell them.

- It's been a bad week for fatigue; couldn't get out of bed at all yesterday, but made it today.

- I know I have to accept these after effects, but it is so hard!

- Some days this stuff gets me more than treatment did. Treatment ended; this won't.

P
is for Personal Philosophy

Sometime during the first couple of weeks of every semester, I ask my students why they enrolled in my Introduction to Philosophy class. Unless they've taken a class from me before, the answer inevitably is: "Because it's required." Now that doesn't exactly warm the cockles of my heart (whatever cockles are), but I know they give me that answer because they haven't a clue what Philosophy is, and they surely don't know that it actually applies to them and represents a sort of skill set that they can use to enhance their lives—give them more meaning and make them more fulfilling. And for us who have survived cancer and its treatment, that's especially important to know!

The word *philosophy* comes from two root words. The first is the Greek, *philos,* meaning loving, and *Sophia,* the goddess of wisdom. So philosophy means loving wisdom, or, to make using it a bit easier, the love of wisdom. I should note here that Sophia was not a goddess in the Greco-Roman pantheon. She was more of an idea, but she is an idea that exists throughout the Western world. Her shrine, Hagia Sophia, located in Istanbul, is one of the Seven Wonders of the World. She is mentioned in all the wisdom books of the Bible, and in parts of the Apocrypha. Solomon, the wisest of kings, was said to have been married to Holy Sophia. Proverbs mentions her, and Ecclesiastes, the teacher, counsels his student to seek her and keep her. We understand, then, that from Egypt to the Celtic people, wisdom was of great value, much greater than mere knowledge, something to seek, find and put into practice throughout one's whole life.

Well, by now you know that Philosophy is my thing. I study it. I teach it. I apply it. I try to live it consciously. I can, given the opportunity, drive people crazy with it. I'll try not to do that to you, though!

Philosophy is the wellspring of all knowledge. It was the first thing people began to do after agriculture was domesticated and there were people who no longer had to spend all their time hunting and gathering to feed their tribal members through the winter. We believe the first philosophers were the wise men or priests within tribal groups. Then the people of Greece began to create city-states, develop political systems for governance and, as they learned to build ships and craft suitable shipping containers, economic systems for trade. As they moved to the great democracy which was the Golden Age of Greece, men who had given up fighting wars began to think about the world around them and wonder how it all came about and what to do next.

The first of these philosophers came from an area known as Miletus, which was located north of Athens. It is so important to keep in mind that when these men began to wonder about things and ask questions about them, there were no universities. There were few books. There was no technology. People travelled throughout the Mediterranean, mostly on foot, and questions and answers travelled with them. They fought wars (of course) and exchanged ideas with those they captured or who captured them, but finally, about 700 years B.C. a group of philosophers had established themselves in Greece.

The first thinker was Thales of Miletus, and his great contribution to wisdom was the identification of the four elements—water, earth, wind and fire. Each philosopher was the mentor of another, and in that way ideas were examined, argued, expanded, accepted or left behind. One of these early philosophers, by the way, was Pythagoras whose Pythagorean Theorem is still used today in geometry classes all over the world.

The important thing for us to know as survivors of cancer and cancer therapies is that we are all living philosophy—usually several of them simultaneously. I promise I won't even try to begin to give you an overview of all the philosophers and their ideas. But what I will do is tell you which philosophers and philosophies influence my thinking and my life, and especially those that helped me through cancer and help me now with long term chemo-brain and other after effects The younger brother, Daniel, of my great-, great-, great-, great-, great-grandmother Hannah Boone was something of a philosopher himself, and he said, "Felicity, the companion of content, is rather found in our own [hearts] than in the enjoyment of external things; and I firmly believe it requires but a little philosophy to make a man happy in whatever state he is". So, I'll follow the advice of Uncle Dan'l, and just give you enough philosophy to help you find felicity.

Plato, which is a nickname that refers to his broad shoulders—he was an Olympic wrestler—is considered the wisest of all philosophers ever. He wrote in the form of dialogues, but he never appeared as a character speaking for himself. Rather, he used his teacher, Socrates, who is considered the first philosopher, as the primary voice in all his work. There are many things about Plato's work that influence me, but the most important for our purposes is his theory of learning. We often hear today that "perception is reality". But Plato would disagree with that mightily. He said perception was just the beginning step on the road to understanding. He laid out a four step process by which a thinker could move from perception, an idea, to opinion, a form of knowledge. But, he said, opinion is the *lowest form of knowledge*. Opinion was just the beginning, and, for the most part, he said, opinions weren't reached by thinking. Rather, they were adopted from someone else, usually someone in authority. (Some things just never change!)

So, I try to follow Plato's philosophy and learn as much as I can about a subject before I decide on my opinion, and I'm always open to changing my opinion if new information becomes available. In the case of this book, for example, after some experience and study, I came to believe (opinion) that some things had changed in me since I first developed cancer and went through treatment. Then with more and more experience and hours and hours of research I found authoritative (Mayo Clinic) support for my idea. And that led to more questions and a whole lot more research from very good authorities, and then I was ready to write a proposal for this book. I had told lots of people that in my opinion I had been permanently affected in some ways by my cancer treatment, and they all pretty much said, "GET OVER IT!" (In terms of opinion, I love to tell the story of a student in one of my university classes who told our professor that she had a right to her opinion, to which he replied quite casually, "And you have a right to remain ignorant". She didn't know her Plato because she didn't stick around after the break!)

In any case, learning everything I could about cancer and its treatment helped me throughout both incidents, helped me develop this book so I could help you, and continues to help me now to cope with what's known and what's not known about the permanent effects of standard chemotherapy. And as far as opinion is concerned, I find I'm a lot like another favorite philosopher, Friedrich Nietzsche, who said, "It is hard enough to remember my opinions, without also remembering my reasons for them!" My students love that.

The second philosopher to influence me was Zeno of Citium. His philosophy is known as Stoicism, and it is based on the idea that everything is one. God is in the earth and in men and men are in the earth and in God, and all things are not just interconnected; they are one. That's an idea that is still popular today and is enjoying a period of new interest and exploration, but the crux of Stoicism is simply this: We must do whatever we can to change unpleasant things so long as there are things we can do; but when there is nothing or nothing more that we can do about the unpleasant thing, we must accept that fact without complaint, because while man does have free will and the ability to act on his choices, all things ultimately rest in the hands of Divine Providence. So, you can clearly see how that would be a philosophy that would help cancer patients and long term survivors. You do everything you can to make it better, and when you've done all you can, you accept the situation and go on. Not an easy philosophy for us 21st century dwellers who tend to be fairly secular in our thinking and think if we just try another angle, we can make the thing work, but Stoicism makes the situation ever so much easier on us when we can do it. You don't give up on a situation; you give in when you've run out of options. When that happens, you have a new situation to work on, and getting stuck in the old one that you can't fix, does no one any good, and, therefore, is not wise.

I've used Immanuel Kant's ethical philosophy throughout this experience. He said that we should only do that which we would make a universal law if we had the power to do so. He said the way to know if what we wanted to do was right was to ask ourselves what it would be like if everyone did what we were thinking of doing. So, after more than a week of listening to another patient complain **daily and unceasingly** about her quarter-sized radiation burn, I did not whip off my gown and show her the deep radiation burn that covered most of one side of my chest! I did not say "You think **you** have a radiation burn? I'll show you a radiation burn!" Nope, I didn't do those things, and Kant would have been proud of me, and my mother laughed until her sides hurt as she imagined my actually doing it!

The Existentialist, Jean Paul Sartre, was a great help because Existentialism says we create our lives by the choices we make. I had to work a bit on the question of whether something I had chosen in the past had created my cancer, but it didn't take much study of Sartre to take care of that notion. Sartre made it clear that the choices we make that create our lives are the ones we make in response to situations that present themselves to us. So, applying Sartre's ideas to my cancer, I made choices as carefully as I could, understanding that the choices I made would affect my life, and if they turned out badly, the resulting circumstances would be mine to deal with without complaint. Sartre said, "It is … senseless to think of complaining since nothing foreign has decided what we feel, what we live, or what we are."

Finally, the last philosopher to help me through my illness and survival is William James, who is fascinating to me because of the ways in which he blended his knowledge of physiology, psychology and philosophy into a pragmatic, sensible philosophy to live by. The famous depth psychologist, Carl Jung, remarked on meeting James and dining with him during a trip Jung made to the United States, and he said it was one of the most interesting and, indeed, delightful evenings of his entire trip. Jung, unlike Freud, allowed for the human soul/spirit, which was something with which James completely agreed. The Pragmatism (the study of the practical/workable) which James developed was very different from that of John Dewey—so much so, in fact, that Dewey changed the name of his philosophy to differentiate it completely from that of James. William James also subscribed to the then relatively new idea of Phenomenology, the idea that you could learn from experience (phenomena). Until Phenomenology was developed in the German school of philosophy, the British idea of Empiricism (accumulated data through scientific experimentation) had ruled Western thinking.

So, we may not know if we love philosophy, but we do for sure live it. And if we can figure out what philosophy we're living and determine if it's really working for us or not, we can have a much better time of it, especially those of us who have been so very sick, and likely will not quite ever be totally well again. We need to make our own philosophical way because as Proust warns us, "Illness is the doctor to whom we pay most heed; to kindness, to knowledge, we make promises only; pain we obey." That's not the way we want to live, is it? Surely, that cannot be the reason we've gone through all this and, to this point at least, survived it. Better, I think, to listen to the Buddha's advice: "To enjoy good health, to bring true happiness to one's family, to bring peace to all, one must first discipline and control one's own mind." Philosophy helps us do that.

Q
is for Quality Survival

Have you seen the movie "The Bucket List" with Jack Nicholson and Morgan Freeman? If you haven't, you really should because it's a charming, entertaining piece that has messages for those of us who have survived cancer. It shows us what the late French surgeon and Nobel prize winner, Alex Carrel, said, "The quality of life is more important than life itself".

In the film, Jack Nicholson (of course) is the leader of the pair, who happen to meet in the cancer ward of a hospital where they both have been diagnosed with terminal disease. The story evolves out of their diagnoses. Nicholson suggests that if he's going to "kick the bucket", then there's a whole list of things he wants to do before that happens. Thus, the bucket list: a list of all those things you want to do before you die. Now, you don't have to have survived cancer to make a bucket list, but if you have, then you certainly should.

My bucket list is not terribly complicated or fancy, but I made it during the first few weeks of my first cancer diagnosis. Here's how my wishes fall, not in any particular order.

*I want to go to Washington, D.C. and the surrounding area.

*I want to go back to New York, and once there I have a sub-list of a whole bunch of things I want to experience again or for the first time.

*I want to see the leaves in New England in the fall—to visit the colors as some say.

*I want to take a course in Philosophy from Dr. Cornell West of Princeton University–I don't care about any grades, although that would be nice to see how I'd do—I just want to be in his space while his mind works.

*A doctorate in consciousness studies at the California Institute for Integral Studies goes on and off my list, but I'm telling you about it because it's not gone altogether yet.

What's on your bucket list? Have you given that any thought? Even if you never had cancer, you should have given some thought to what you wanted to do before you "kick the bucket". But in our culture, we're taught to be practical and not think about foolish things like a small Italian restaurant in Greenwich Village in Manhattan or unnecessary things for ordinary people like an opera at the Metropolitan Opera or a day at that Museum of Modern Art or the Metropolitan, or a live play on Broadway or even off-Broadway, or a visit to the World Trade Center Memorial or a show at Carnegie Hall—all in Manhattan. If we have been fortunate enough to survive cancer, especially if we've survived for several years, the practical goal is to get back to normal as soon as possible. Normal, of course, means that we should try to act like nothing happened. But normal isn't normal for us anymore. We understand that what we call "normal" can be tossed upside-down, inside-out and backwards in the blink of an eye! Hummingbirds can't fly as fast as "normal" can just plain disappear. And we also know now that life is short, and if we don't make plans to do what we want to do, we may never get the chance.

It seems to me we are all trained to believe what Robert Fulghum wrote in his book All I Need to Know I Learned in Kindergarten: "Beware of wonder" he said. "Live a balanced life - learn some and think some and draw and paint and sing and dance and play and work every day some." I can't believe how much I agreed with him when I read that. But that was before I went to college and before I got my first cancer. Now I agree with Mark Twain, who said, "Twenty years from now you will be more disappointed by the things that you didn't do than by the ones you did do. So throw off the bowlines. Sail away from the safe harbor. Catch the trade winds in your sails. Explore. Dream. Discover". I'm going to tell you a story in a little bit which never would have happened in my life if I had taken Fulghum's advice to "beware of wonder". Now I love the experience of wonder, and I search it out so I can add things to my bucket list.

I am a political junkie and have been as long as I can remember. I've been saying for years that it is not acceptable that someone who is as political as I am should not see Washington, D. C. Now, though, it's on my bucket list. In three years my sister and I are going to Washington, and then on to New York, and then on to New England. We are making plans because "someday" may never come. We'll fly East and join a group to stay in a hostel in D,C, When we've covered as much of the Washington area as we want to see, it will be Amtrak to New York City and when we're done there, a rental car into the northeast. The more we plan, the more real the adventure seems.

I used to go to New York on business every year, and the year I started college, I spent an afternoon at the Museum of Modern Art, having decided to put into practice the advice of the ancient Greek, Herodotus, who said "All men's gains are the fruit of venturing." And I was venturing out on something new that day; I had never been in a museum because I was always working. But that semester I had taken a course in art history and was determined to see some of the real thing after viewing a whole term of slides. And what a day it was! I saw Vincent Van Gogh's "Starry Night", and it is a glorious little painting. For years I had seen Jasper Johns' "Flag" in books and magazines, and thought "Anyone could do that. You need some red, white and blue paint and a ruler." And then I saw the painting itself, and I was amazed. Johns' painting is a collage. The American flag is painted on a mid-sized canvas which is covered with copies of the New York Times. The painting is not a flag; it's a visual manifestation of the idea of freedom of speech. It's a painting of the First Amendment to the Constitution, and I never would have known that if I hadn't decided I would by golly go to that museum. But Van Gogh and Johns, as wonderful as they were, were just the beginning.

As I moved through the museum, enjoying some pieces, curious about others, and completely turned off by others, I noticed an alcove off to my left just ahead of me. I turned into that space, having not the slightest idea of what I would see, and it was a very good thing there was an empty bench very close by. Otherwise, I'd have been on the floor, because my knees went right out from under me. In that alcove was a triptych of Claude Monet's "Water Lilies". The painting consists of three panels, each eight feet tall by fourteen feet wide. The painting is of the lily pond on Monet's farm in France, which he painted many times in many forms. But the size of this rendering was just overwhelming, and for me it was a spiritual experience in that I realized for the first time in my life what the human soul is capable of bringing into being! It still takes my breath away when I think of it.

And I want to do that again. And I want my sister, who is an artist, to do it with me. And so it is on my bucket list, and we are making plans. In the meantime, I go to museums and art exhibitions as often as I can, and I have put together a small collection of original art that brings me great joy every day. I wouldn't have any of that if I had stuck with "normal".

And here's just a little aside that you can use whenever you think of a bucket list item and tell yourself you can't do it. When Monet painted this huge masterpiece, he was over 80 years old, nearly blind, and his assistants had to tape the paint brushes to his hands because he had such severe arthritis. If Monet could do that and create such magnificence, you can make a bucket list, and you can do the things you put on it!

Thoreau tells us, "Do not lose hold of your dreams or aspirations. For if you do, you may still exist but you will have ceased to live". But your bucket list isn't about dreams or even aspirations. It's about intention and plans and determination and will. It's about living the wisdom Eleanor Roosevelt expressed, when she said, "The purpose of life, after all, is to live it, to taste experience to the utmost, to reach out eagerly and without fear for newer and richer experience". You survived cancer to do that!

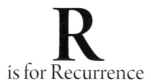

R

is for Recurrence

I'm not sure when I started reading the obituaries in our local newspaper before I read the front page, but I know it was after my first cancer. I still do it… I don't pay much attention to anyone over age 80 or so, I look for younger women, and I search for cancer as a cause of death or a request for donations to Hospice in lieu of flowers. And I'll bet I'm not alone in this rather morbid activity! I always say a little prayer for the one we lost, and I remember one that said the woman had passed after a 14 year battle with breast cancer. Fourteen years!! Good for her! The most interesting one I've seen so far was one that said the woman won her battle with cancer when she died. I still think about that one. If we were using a sports metaphor, I think that would at best be a forfeit, but I'm not sure.

So here I am after all these years, writing about cancer deaths and recurrences and other not-so-happy things we sometimes think about. But think about them we do, so we have to talk about them here. I'd like to think that the further away I get from diagnosis and am still cancer free, the less I would think about a recurrence. But that's not the way it goes. Just a few months ago, Dr. P looked at me and said, "No one is ever going to be able to convince you that it's not coming back are they", and I immediately responded with a negative shaking of my head. Nope. Not even after all these years. I don't ever think about a recurrence of my ovarian cancer, but every now and then I still think about a return of the breast cancer. We all know there is no cure for breast cancer, although survival rates are up so dramatically and so many of us are surviving for so much longer after treatment. But there is no cure. The further away we get from diagnosis the lower the odds of a recurrence go. But there is no cure. Not yet. And we know that.

Now the interesting thing is that my response—and most likely yours— is not unusual. In fact, every study of cancer survivors' fears of recurrence, especially with breast cancer, tells us that the length of survival time at the time of the psychological testing makes no difference. A study by Crespi, et al, published in the Journal of the National Cancer Institute in 2008 states, "a number of studies (citing sources) have shown that long-term cancer survivors have fairly high levels of functioning on generic measures of health-related quality of life, However, a large [body of] literature indicates that the experiences of cancer diagnosis, treatment, **and survival** can engender lingering problems and concerns across physical psychological, social and spiritual dimensions" (emphasis added). Imagine that; the very experience of surviving can play a part in recurrence anxiety! I'm not really surprised, though, because I think all of us who have had cancer are always afraid in the far back of our minds that it's going to come and bite us again. It's the bogey man under the bed, the home invasion robber and the thief that comes in the night all rolled into one. And it's a well-known serial killer that preys on men and women alike, so we'd be silly to just ignore the possibility that it might come back.

But the news from the world of science is not all bad. That same study goes on to report that "The experience of long-term survivorship can include positive life changes as well, such as personal growth (citing sources), an increased sense of meaning or purpose (citing sources) and positive effects on relationships (citing sources)."

All of this work on quality of life for long-term survivors is very valuable on many levels, but it does worry me some. Now make no mistake; I don't know anything about preparing a scientific study. I had to take statistics in graduate school, but my professor's philosophy was that we needed more to know how to interpret statistics than to create them. He figured if we went on to do a thesis that required statistical analysis, we could hire him to help us do it. Now that's a practical professor! So my questions about the fear studies don't have anything to do with their numbers. My concern is with the words they use and their failure to define them. Let me show you what I mean.

I found a 2007 study published in *Health and Quality of Life Outcomes* that reported on a newly developed questionnaire that could be used to measure the experience. The researchers had a good sample that included both short and long term survivors, but they used a number of terms to define the feelings of their subjects, and that concerns me. Socrates said we couldn't really have a complete discussion until we defined for everyone what we were talking about, and that's my problem here. To say that I won't ever be convinced my cancer won't return is not to say that I worry about it or even think of it often. To say that I worry about it is not to say that I'm concerned about it. To admit I'm not convinced it will never come back doesn't mean that I'm afraid it will. And then to embrace all of this with the phrase "significant negative psychological consequences" is, I think, dangerous.

Before I found proof that my current symptoms were associated with my cancer treatment, I experienced a number of negative psychological states, frustration being first among them. When we couldn't identify any reasons for the way I felt, I would certainly wonder if it could be cancer again that we just couldn't find. But to wonder or question is not to worry or be concerned. And so my worry involves the fact that we live in a time of medication for all things, especially all things psychological. I sometimes take an SSRI for short periods, as I've said before. But it took a very long time for us to decide I should do that. We were and are extremely careful with my medications, and I don't take anything we aren't both sure I need, and even then we watch everything very carefully.

So I can't help but wonder how many survivors have been diagnosed as depressed or anxious or some other "negative psychological" state and are taking medication they don't need because their problems are really a matter of long term after effects of chemotherapy and other cancer treatment. How many are resigned to having psychological issues because they're tired of appearing to "cry wolf" all the time? For many folks it must be a lot better to have *some* explanation, even if it's not the right one.

And so, we need to take these worries, concerns, constant fears, and fearful psychological constructs in hand and ask for a thorough evaluation of our psychological status as well as our long term effects of cancer therapy. If we are part of the potentially very high percentage of cancer survivors whose brains have been affected by chemotherapeutic agents, then we can't even know how psychotropic medications will affect us. We don't know if they are safe for us, which is why they must be monitored so carefully. And, unfortunately, we are all too willing in our country these days to accept a diagnosis of a mental illness. I can't begin to tell you how many of my students are taking psychotherapeutic drugs for their "issues", and their brains aren't even formed yet!

Oops! Let me get down off my high horse, I got carried away there for just a little bit. But I am passionate about this brain stuff. We only have one of those, and it has to last us a lifetime because transplantation of that organ hasn't yet been figured out. And we know now that a potentially huge number of cancer patients have incurred injury to their brains as a result of the cancer treatment. Primary care docs, oncologists, neurologists and psychologists all have to be made aware of these new findings about the potential damage caused to the patient's central nervous system by cancer treatment so that they can develop plans of treatment that really meet the needs of the patient who, after all, would like to have a high quality of life after having been through the anguish of cancer.

Finally, what do we do if we do have a recurrence? In an article entitled "When Cancer Returns: How to Cope with Cancer Recurrence", published by the Mayo Clinic in 2011, a recurrence is described as a cancer that returns after a period of remission. The Mayo staff tells us that recurrence is divided into three categories. A local recurrence is one where the cancer reappears where it was first found or in a nearby place and has not spread to lymph nodes or other body parts. A regional recurrence is found in the lymph nodes and tissue in the general area of the original cancer. And a distant recurrence is one that has spread or metastasized to a part of the body that is at a distance from the original cancer.

Mayo's report says that in the case of most cancers, a local recurrence may still be curable, but the odds for a cure of a distant recurrence are not good. Treatment for recurrences is, of course, available. Even if the cancer can't be beaten again, treatments are available that may shrink the tumor or slow the growth of the cancer. These treatments can relieve pain and other symptoms and extend your life. That's when decisions have to be made taking into account the factors involved in your original cancer, the treatment you received and your responses to it, how many and what kind of side effects would be involved in the new treatment and your willingness to endure them. And you cannot know any of those things unless and until a recurrence appears.

So, that's what I think about when I think about a possible recurrence of my cancer. I wonder if I would go through treatment again, knowing what I know now and assuming my team would be willing to treat me. That's the only thing I question myself about. And since I can't decide that now, there's nothing much to think about. Certainly there is nothing now to worry about or concern myself with or become anxious or depressed about. If I were to experience those negative emotions in connection with recurrence fears, I would absolutely see a therapist.

But now, since I don't have those negative emotional states to deal with, when the notion of a recurrence does come to mind, I rely on the wisdom of the ancients, which is the way of a philosopher (and everyone is a philosopher). I like what Chuang Tzu, a follower of Lao Tzu, said in the 4th century BC. He said, "Accept whatever happens, and let your spirit move freely". And if a worst case scenario were to arise for me, I'd like to think I would rely on the advice of the ancient Greek philosopher, Pythagoras (yes, he of the triangles), who said, "Choose rather to be strong of soul than strong of body". That's really all I can do.

S
is for Spirituality

Over the years I've come to believe that spirituality is in my blood. My paternal great-grandfather was a circuit riding preacher in Oregon during the Gold Rush era. My maternal uncle was a priest in the Church of England. My older sister is an ordained minister in the United Church of Christ, and my younger sister and I both teach religious studies. There's got to be something genetic in there somewhere, don't you think? I think this quote from Dante Gabriel Rossetti, a 19th century poet and artist is both humorous and true: "The worst moment for the atheist is when he is really thankful and has nobody to thank"! And we who are long term survivors of cancer have plenty to be thankful for, even the opportunity to be the first to make our way through these sometimes awful after effects of our treatment.

The word "religion" comes from the Latin word, *religio* which means to reconnect, to link back. So what do we reconnect or link back to? Well, that depends on your traditions, your theology, your own cosmology or world view. While we can subscribe to the prescriptions of a specific religion or theology, we don't have to. While we can abide by the rules of a specific church or mosque or temple, we don't have to. We don't even have to be limited by a certain view of the Divine Energy. We don't have to think of the Divine as an old man with a long white beard. That's Zeus! All religions agree that the Divine has no attributes, that is, no physical presence as we understand it, at all. Some people make images to represent certain aspects of the Divine, and the three Western religions—Judaism, Christianity and Islam, all worshiping the same God—are directed in scripture not even to try to make an image of the Creator.

If we don't have or choose to follow a set of other manmade rules, we can always rely on the ideas of Aristotle. He believed that the world came into being somehow, although he could not explain it any more than anyone can today. But obviously Aristotle knew the world existed because he was in it. He knew it had to come from somewhere, and he could see that it "operates". It goes from night to day, it moves from one season to another, and all things come into being and ultimately fade away. So, he (the father of logic) determined that once the world was created by whatever means, there had to be some sort of energy that got everything going, and he called that the Prime Mover.

None of us can know for sure about anything concerning religion except that it appears always to have existed in human experience, at least in terms of a belief in some mysterious "other" from which we come and to which we return. So, what we connect to, what we relink to, I think, is our Selves. "We can no more do without spirituality than we can do without food, shelter, or clothing" wrote the late Ernest Holmes (1887-1960), an American minister, philosopher and author of *Science of the Mind*, and I find that to be true. I found it especially to be true when I went through cancer treatments.

While my "little" self (body-ego) went about doing what had to be done to fight my cancers, teach my students and help my mom, my Self was busy keeping my spirit connected to that which cannot be known. My Self needed courage, so I thought often about my great-, great-, great-, great-, great-grandmother's younger brother, Daniel Boone. That was one courageous guy! In one letter he said, "I was happy in the midst of dangers and inconveniences". I can imagine wandering around the wilds of Kentucky was darned dangerous and inconvenient, but so is chemotherapy! So I thought about the fact that I was a many generations later child of the same blood as Daniel Boone, and I'd think how heroic he was and the need for heroism of a different kind in facing cancer and its treatment, and I could relate to my ancestor.

As the side effects of treatment began to set in, and I lost the rest of the hair I hadn't shaved off, and my memory for names especially began to fail me, and the second time around when I begged Dr. Alali to let me stop, I could once again connect with my famous uncle, who said, "I have never been lost, but I will admit to being confused for several weeks". For me, that described my response to both episodes of cancer and cancer treatment perfectly. I never lost my Self, but I was often very confused.

I tried then, and I try even now, not to worry too much. When a new symptom presents itself, you can't really stop yourself from thinking about what that might be. But as Mahatma Gandhi, who suffered bodily abuse and the pain of self-imposed fasting for his cause tells us, "There is nothing that wastes the body like worry." For us who have suffered through and survived cancer and its treatment, that is very good advice. If we worry, we are draining our bodies of the strength they need to survive and then to keep on living despite the toxins they have absorbed.

I often use Bible phrases to keep my Self grounded and away from worry, and I'll share them with you. I especially like, "Be still and know that

I am God" from Psalm 46. I also like this from the 121ˢᵗ Psalm, which I have personalized: "I lift up my eyes to the hills, from where my help comes. My help comes from the Lord, and He will not let my foot be moved. The Lord is the shade at my right hand, and He will keep my life". "Thy will, not mine" is a constant in my mind, as is "Thank you", which I try to remember to say for every gift, even a parking place in a crowded lot—nothing is too small to be thankful for, I think! "Be here now" comes from the title of a book by Baba Ram Dass, which was published in 1971 and which I still keep at the ready.

I think everything that comes to us is an opportunity to learn, so I try very hard to find the lesson in every experience, and discover how I can work it into my life. All of that is, of course, a matter of consciousness, and ever since my university studies of consciousness from an interdisciplinary standpoint, I have realized how easy it is to fall into a passive, numb state where you are aware of nothing but the puny surface matters of your life. I tell students that I don't believe anyone on their death bed ever says, "I sure wish I'd spent more time at the office"!

I have a few things that I keep in sight so that I can remember to reconnect to my Self. I have pictures of my mother and father, my grandparents and my aunts to remind my Self that I come from a line of people who lived, loved, struggled and suffered just as I have—perhaps not under exactly the same circumstances, but certainly under circumstances no less difficult for them. I have my mother's little bronzed baby shoes on the table by my bed, so I see them every morning. I have luncheon plates in my china cabinet that were hand painted by my mother and by her mother to remind me that my people are creative, and creativity is an act of worship in my view. I have my great-, great-, great-grandmother's wooden mixing bowl and her rolling pin that has only one handle because she wore one of them away. She brought those with her in a covered wagon from Nebraska, and when I use them, I am almost one with her in spirit. And, of course, I have my copy of the family tree that proves that I am a descendant of Hannah Boone, sister of Daniel.

I also have a small collection of original art, believing as I do with Schopenhauer, that true peace can be found in nature, music and art. I have three paintings done by my sister at various times in her life as an artist. One, an abstract she titled "Missions" has been with me for more than 35 years and has always been in a prominent place in my living room where I can see it whenever I'm at home and awake. I have another abstract done by an artist in Humboldt County between the time she was diagnosed with cancer and the beginning of her chemo, which was going to occur the day after I bought her painting. I am honored to have it.

I have landscapes of the valley in which I live, watercolors most of them, and they remind me that I and my Self are here where my people have been since before the Gold Rush. One piece of art that I own is very popular with friends and family alike. It's a winter scene of bare birch trees in the snow, and I really enjoy people's comments because it is a nicely framed 50 cent poster! So art is available to us all.

Books are my true passion; I'm never without one. Film is important, but a live stage performance is even better for the spirit. I worry for my students that they so limit their own exposure to the arts, and our school systems are so short-sighted and so short on funding that many of them are unable to provide musical study as they did in my youth. As far as I'm concerned, the spiritual life requires the Native American flute, the Mormon Tabernacle Choir, the Harlem Gospel Choir, Tibetan Buddhist chanting, a good symphony orchestra and Yo-Yo Ma. If the Self gets a fair supply of those things, the self can handle a bit of rap!

The life of the Self, the essence of our Being, need not be dull or boring or expensive to maintain. To bring that essence into Being requires only consciousness, openness, intention and determination. The 20th century's greatest scientist, we nearly all agree, was Albert Einstein. He said, "All religions, arts and sciences are branches of the same tree", and that's an authority we can rely on if anyone questions our new efforts at exploring our Selves and our lives.

I want to leave this chapter on spirituality with a quote from one of my very favorite actors and activists for peace, Martin Sheen: "… I think that [the] basic foundation of faith is personal conscience. I think it's between you and God, not you and the Church." I agree.

T
is for Teeth

I have my father's teeth. Well, not literally, of course, but when my personal zygote was swimming around in the gene pool, it picked up the blend of soft enamel and strong roots that runs in the teeth of my paternal line. So I have spent more than my share of time in a dentist's chair. But I have been reassured by every dentist I've ever seen that my never ending cavities were not really a problem because the important part of teeth is the roots, and I had exceptional roots. A good dentist can repair the external parts of the teeth, they said, but if the roots aren't solid, then you really can have problems. What they didn't know, though, was what chemotherapy and radiation can do to those choppers, no matter how strong the roots have always been.

And I have to remind myself that they didn't know; that before any after effect can really be considered a long term effect of cancer treatment, enough of us have to survive long enough for the after effect to develop, and then it takes a while for enough of us to think the problem is related to cancer or to cancer treatment, and then enough of us have to report the problem, and then someone can finally get to work on it. That applies to every after effect I talk about in this book.

Of those, dental problems might well be the most difficult and expensive of all the after effects of cancer therapy. People often say the worst part of chemotherapy is losing your hair, but I can attest to the fact that after you've survived the treatment and your tresses have regrown to some extent, losing your teeth is a whole lot more traumatic--and expensive!

The Mayo Clinic has verified these dental problems can appear and continue long after your cancer treatment has ended. There is not much evidence to tell us why it happens, but there is no doubt that cancer treatment can result in dental cavities and infections, and I have found no insurance that covers the expense involved. In fact, when my oncologist suggested my own reconstructions should be covered by my medical insurance because they were a result of my cancer treatment, I discovered that my policy specifically denies coverage for dental work related to cancer treatment. (I guess someone knew there could be problems!)

The first hint I had that dental problems could arise from cancer treatment came while I was waiting to begin chemo the first time, and I found one short reference from the National Institutes of Health regarding a need for custom made trays into which you would place fluoride gel and wear for about half an hour each day to protect the teeth.

Since that first hint from the National Institutes of Health, I've lately found a few more fairly well hidden, brief references to dental problems developing as a result of cancer treatment, but they are few and far between, although the Mayo Clinic acknowledges the problem. Some say that radiation is the bad actor behind dental cavities and infections, and that you only need to worry about your teeth if you had radiation to the head and neck. Others say it's the combination of chemotherapy and radiation that causes the problems. But even though the specific aspect of treatment that causes the problems is uncertain, the problems can develop and do exist, and they are serious.

When teeth become infected, they may have to be extracted or root-canaled or crowned. If extractions are necessary, those teeth will have to be replaced by dentures or implants, or crowns and complicated bridgework. I've had all those things—more than once—and you might well wonder why I don't just get false teeth and be done with it. Well, that's because every one of those dentists I've seen over my life has pointed out that dentures are not possible for me. And it may be that you won't be able just to get false teeth either because your mouth, like mine, might not be able to accommodate them. And, on top of that, everyone agrees on one thing: Your own teeth are always better than dentures.

As experienced as I am in matters dental, I still agree completely with Johnny Depp when he says, "Trips to the dentist--I like to postpone that kind of thing." But if you've survived cancer treatment, you can't postpone that trip for very long. If you do, you might just find out that you've bitten off more than you can chew! (pun intended)

My first total dental reconstruction became necessary about four years after my first cancer and its treatment. After that was completed I followed Johnny Depp's advice for a couple of years, but when I lost a crown, I couldn't delay my appointment any longer. And soon I found myself in the dentist's recliner for up to six or seven hours at a time in circumstances much less comfortable than a chemotherapy infusion center! At least, though, having now spent enough on my teeth to pay for a mid-sized car, I finally have my fluoride trays! I hope it won't take ten years for you to get yours!

And there are other things you can do, as well. One of the major problems that chemotherapy brings is dry mouth, which is a major cause of dental cavities and infections. Like so many other side effects of chemotherapy, the general assumption has been that the side effect of dry mouth would end when the treatment ended, but the truth is, it doesn't. So hydration is very important. Dry, flaky (not chapped) lips are an indication that we're not getting enough fluid, so it's good to drink lots of water and other non-sugared drinks. There is also a product line called Biotene which you can find in the dental supplies aisle of your drug or grocery store. Biotene helps with the dry mouth problem, but doesn't resolve it completely. I use the toothpaste and mouthwash and carry mouth spray with me to use during the day, and it helps. Biotene products are a bit more expensive than the average toothpaste, but compared to the price of a gold crown, they're a real bargain!

Keeping teeth immaculately clean is also crucial for the cancer patient who has survived treatment. Brushing at least twice a day, but preferably after every meal, is absolutely necessary. A regular toothbrush is really not enough to assure the complete cleaning that we need, so if you don't have an electric brush, you should invest in one. I recommend the Oral B electric toothbrush, distributed by Proctor & Gamble. We who do have post cancer treatment dental problems need the model that has the clock and three speeds (high, low and massage) because it does all the brushing, assures that every area of the mouth is evenly covered and does it all with the gentle action that protects the gums. I had been told from the time of my first crown that gentle brushing of the gums was important. When I had the first reconstruction, the specialist said I needed to be "scrubbing" fluoride gel into my gum line. Then when I met my new dentist, she said "Oh, you're brushing too hard." Sometimes, to paraphrase the actress, Helen Hayes, I am confused by life, and feel safe only in the confines of the classroom. (For Ms. Hayes, the safe place was the theater.)

But there is no confusion about the need for flossing! Flossing is necessary after every meal. If you have permanent bridges, use floss threaders to get under them. Use dental picks if you're out in public, but you still have to floss thoroughly when you get home.

So the instructions are basically the same as those for a six year old: brush, brush, brush—but gently, please. Use toothpaste and mouth wash formulated to reduce dry mouth—never use mouthwash containing alcohol which is very drying. Do fluoride soaks every day, and have your teeth cleaned by your dentist every three months—four times a year, not two.

That's the only advice I have, and it comes to you at great expense in every way that can be imagined when it comes to dental work. But don't follow it if you don't want to. You can, if you want, go with the humorist, S. J. Perlman, who said, "I'll dispose of my teeth as I see fit, and after they've gone, I'll get along. I started off living on gruel, and by God, I can always go back to it again." Before I made that decision, though, I'd want to have a preview taste of that gruel!

U
is for Useful

I just have to ask: If you hadn't survived, what would they have said about you? What would you want them to have said about you? Would they have said your life had meaning? Would they have said you contributed something with your life? Would they have said that despite your battle against cancer you gave your all to making your life and the lives of others better and more worthwhile? Would they say you took the advice of the 20th century philosopher, James Allen, to "Above all be of single aim; have a legitimate and useful purpose, and devote yourself unreservedly to it"?

The one thing cancer survivors always hear is that we must do something with the lives that have been given us. Well, I think everyone ought to do that, but I agree it's very important for us. We need to know that we survived for a reason. We need to find the reason and live it.

We cannot kid ourselves. We have suffered through this miserable disease, but Friedrich Nietzsche, who is one of my very favorite thinkers, said this about suffering: "To live is to suffer; to survive is to find some meaning in the suffering". So survival isn't just a matter of keeping on breathing when the treatment is done. Survival involves finding something to have survived for, a reason for having survived when so many others have not.

I tell students that I think I survived cancer so that I could stick around and annoy them. They're not sure whether to believe me or not! But I do think teaching, and especially teaching philosophy, has been the purpose of my life and the thing that has brought real meaning to it. It's a nerve-wracking business. I never know if they "get it" when I'm teaching it. I'm constantly evaluating my presentations and my approaches to make sure I'm staying on task. And it's a lot of work! But one of the things that keeps me going is the fact that although they might not get it now, I don't know that they won't get it later. I am always assured that there may very well come a point at some time in their future when they need to make a wise choice, and they will say, "Oh, that's what Professor Wheeler meant!" As frustrated as I sometimes get, as worried as I often get, I know without a single doubt that I am making their lives better for them, even if they don't know it now.

I have also come to believe that I survived two cancers in order to experience the long term effects of treatment, especially chemotherapy, so that I could search for and find the truth about what it means to be a cancer patient—once a cancer patient, always a cancer patient—and write this book for you and your medical providers. And my hope in accomplishing that task is the same as my hope for my students: that you will be able to say about some pain or sense of discomfort that you experience, "Oh, that's what that woman was saying in her book!"

The famous Russian writer, Leo Tolstoy, wrote that the "sole meaning of life is to serve humanity", and that's what I hope I do. Plato said that man is a being in search of meaning, and he is considered one of the wisest men ever to have lived. So I have to ask you if you are searching for meaning in your life as a survivor. You aren't the same, you know, as you were before the cancer. You just can't go through all that without being changed. Given that fact, the question to be asked is, what is your purpose now? How will you bring meaning to this life that you and your team have worked so hard to keep on land?

C. S. Lewis, the great English author of "The Lion, the Witch and the Wardrobe" as well as the entire Narnia series and a number of books on Christianity, to which he came quite late in life, believed that reason is the order of truth, but imagination is the organ of meaning. So what are you imagining, not only for yourself, but for everyone who could use something that you have to give? In the chapter on Quality we talked about things you'd like to do, and that takes quite a lot of imagination. But this question takes even more.

This question takes imagination and courage and a willingness to make mistakes in your efforts to create meaning. Freud's protégé, Carl Jung, believed that a least little thing with meaning is worth more in one's life than the greatest things that have no meaning. The imagination that Lewis talks about is very close to curiosity, a characteristic that is all too often missing in our busy, hectic, structured lives today. You know, when our children begin to talk we are so excited and we encourage them and chatter back with them, and that's how they learn language. The brain is fascinating in the way it takes in language when children are little. And we are so very proud of our little ones as they struggle to learn words. At least we are right up until they learn the word, "why". Now that's a whole different story! If only we would learn to ask them what they think the answer to their question is, both our lives would be easier, and we could say as Eleanor Roosevelt did, "…at a child's birth, if a mother could ask a fairy godmother to endow it with the most useful gift, that gift would be curiosity". Curiosity about yourself and the world around you, combined with unbridled imagination, can lead your child to a meaningful life, as it can lead you to a new, more complete meaning in your new life as a survivor.

And there is so much to do! In these days of budget cuts at every level, everybody needs help, individuals and organizations. The various cancer organizations need volunteers, support groups need speakers, lonely people need company, teachers need classroom help with ever larger classes, youth groups need mentors to guide teens through tough times. It just goes on and on. And if you work at a job, too, then finding time to make meaning in your life will not be easy. But if you go back to my chapter on Energy, you'll remember there are ways to get it done!

You must remember, though, not to make the things you do to make your life more meaningful just another job—more work. When you find this thing only you can contribute, it must be of greater value to you than anyone else. I know it sounds trite, but you really must feel called to do it. The wonderful writer, Evelyn Underwood, said "Deliberately seek opportunities for kindness, sympathy, and patience". Nothing could be better than that. The Asian goddess, Quan Yin, is known as the Goddess of Mercy, and it is said that she lived such a kind and compassionate life that she became clear and was qualified to enter Nirvana. But just as she approached the gate, she heard the cries of distress from the earth below, and she turned away from paradise to return to the earth as a Bodhisattva, one who helps others along their rocky path. Quan Yin is deeply loved in Chinese Buddhism because "she who was born of the lotus" is the archetypal model of gentle, nurturing feminine love.

And when you have put forth the effort to find the thing or things that will bring greater depth and meaning and wonder to your life, you will be like St. Basil's tree. "A tree is known by its fruit", he said, "a man by his deeds. A good deed is never lost; he who sows courtesy reaps friendship, and he who plants kindness gathers love."

In "The Bucket List", one of the characters says to the other, "You know, the ancient Egyptians had a beautiful belief about death. When their souls got to the entrance to heaven, the guards asked two questions. Their answers determined whether they were able to enter or not. 'Have you found joy in your life?' 'Has your life brought joy to others?'"

If you could give a positive answer to both of those questions, you couldn't possibly have led a better life or had any more worthwhile reason to have survived your cancer.

V

is for Voices of Others

In previous chapters I've given you lots of hints and ideas about what kept me going through cancer and its treatment as well as what keeps me going as I deal with the after effects of chemotherapy. Here I'd like to give you some things from other people and sources, some known and others unknown, that appeal to me and that I think you might find helpful as well. I think there's something here for every state of mind you might experience on this path. I found these first poems online:

Have You Ever Wondered Why
Have you ever wondered why it was her and not me?
The girl who was nice, was good, was sweet
The one who would honor, forgive and forget
Why her and not me, she is such a delight
Her suffering and pain, her fear and her doubts
Why her and not me, she doesn't deserve pain
Her beauty and grace, her compassion and joy
Why her and not me, life is so...............why?
Anonymous

Dreams
I look to the sky and what do I see?
A castle, a rainbow, and dreams for me,
An end to this battle that I must fight,
It will be here someday... someday.
Anonymous

Slow Dance

Have you ever watched kids on a merry-go-round?
Or listened to the rain slapping on the ground?
Ever followed a butterfly's erratic flight?

Or gazed at the sun into the fading night?
You better slow down, don't dance so fast.
Time is short and the music won't last.

Do you run through each day on the fly?
When you ask "How are you?" do you hear the reply?
When the day is done do you lie in your bed
With the next hundred chores running thru your head?
You'd better slow down, don't dance so fast.
Time is short and the music won't last.

Ever told your child we'll do it tomorrow?
And in your haste, not seen his sorrow?
Ever lost touch, let a good friendship die
Cause you never had time to call and say "Hi"?
You'd better slow down, don't dance so fast.
Time is short, and the music won't last.

When you run so fast to get somewhere
You miss half the fun of being there.
When you worry and hurry through your day,
It's like an unopened gift....thrown away.

Life is not a race.
Do take it slower.
Hear the music before the song is over.

Anonymous

This next exclamation comes from a young woman who is four years out of treatment. She shared her thoughts online: "I beat you 4 years ago. But the depression has never [gone] away and now I have to deal with the horrible side effects you and the treatments left behind. Why did I have to deal with you and fight for my life? Why do I have to live in fear you will come back?"

When I studied religion at the university, I came to know the writings of a Cistercian monk whose secular name was Thomas Merton. There is nothing I wouldn't read if it were written by Thomas Merton, and I really recommend his first book, a sort of forced autobiography, entitled "Seven Storey

Mountain". Merton's writing is elegant, and his personal story, and his later writings on peace, Bible stories, and the similarities among religions are just inspiring. This poem by Merton will help anyone stand strong with courage as they deal with cancer and its after effects.

> MY LORD GOD,
> I have no idea where I am going.
> I do not see the road ahead of me.
> I cannot know for certain where it will end.
> Nor do I really know myself, and the fact that I think that
> I am following your will does not mean that I am actually
> doing so.
> But I believe that the desire to please you does in fact
> please you.
> And I hope I have that desire in all that I am doing.
> I hope that I will never do anything apart from that desire.
> And I know that if I do this you will lead me by the right
> road though I may know nothing about it. Therefore will I
> trust you always though I may seem to be lost and in the
> shadow of death.
> I will not fear, for you are ever with me, and you will never
> leave me to face my perils alone.

There just isn't anyone like Merton as far as I'm concerned, and another thing on my personal bucket list is to visit the Abbey at Louisville, Kentucky just to walk on the same ground that he did. Perhaps we can go there on our way home from "leaf peeping".

I find a great deal of comfort and wisdom in the wisdom of the Eastern writers, as well. One of my favorite books is the "Tao de Ching" by Lao Tzu, which means "old man". The story goes that Lao Tzu had been trying to teach the people how to live in harmony with the earth and with each other for many years, but he had no luck. The people were as jealous and greedy and angry after he spoke as before. So, it's said, he finally gave up. He made up his mind to leave the city and go into the forest to live the life of a hermit. In those days all the cities were surrounded by high walls to protect the residents from invaders, and, of course, the walls were guarded. It's said that when Lao Tzu approached the gate, the young man on guard duty asked where he was going. Lao Tzu replied that he was tired of trying to teach the people the right way to live, nobody listened to him, and he was tired of wasting his time. The young man was wiser than his years because he begged the old man to write down his teachings so the people would at least have them if they woke up one day. Reluctantly (I think) Lao Tzu wrote down 81 very brief chapters, and then went on his way to solitude. One of my favorite verses is Chapter Six, called The Mysterious Female

> The Valley Spirit never dies.
> It is named the Mysterious Female.
> And the doorway of the Mysterious Female
> Is the sea from which Heaven and Earth sprang.
> It is there within us all the while;
> Draw upon it as you will, it never runs dry.

The feminine principle that Lao Tzu refers to is the everlasting nurturing, comforting, gentle and compassionate universal energy that offers kindness to all who look for it. Here's another chapter from "The Tao" which helps me along:

> Simplicity, patience, compassion.
> These three are your greatest treasures....
> Compassionate toward yourself,
> You reconcile all beings in the world.

I found two short lines in a little book called "The Choice is Always Ours" by Dorothy Phillips, Elizabeth Howes and Lucille Nixon, all Jungian therapists. These two little lines seem to me to hold one in good stead if they're used as sort of a mantra. The first comes from John Donne: "Affliction is a treasure...that makes us fit for God". The second is from Frances G. Wickes: "You must strip yourself of all self-deception". That's a slightly stronger version of Socrates' statement in his closing argument to the jury that charged him with corrupting the youth of Athens. He just said, "Know thyself, for the unexamined life is not worth living". When I'm dealing with cancer, Donne and Wickes get more attention from me than Socrates!

The English poet, W. H Auden, offers wisdom in the second line of "For the Time Being". He said, "The distresses of choice are our chance to be blessed". I was very happy when I found this one because one of the things I teach my young students is that free will is not a gift; it is a burden! We have to be responsible for our choices and their outcomes. Needless to say, my students don't like it when I tell them that (and I tell them fairly often) because they like the idea of having the freedom to choose, which at their age they interpret as meaning the freedom to do as they please. (When you're dealing with cancer, hanging around a bunch of young college students also makes it easier to learn patience!)

I love this quote about his cancer, which was published in the January, 2012 issue of "Vanity Fair" in an interview with the reporter and writer, Christopher Hitchens, who passed away soon after: "So far, I have decided to take whatever my disease can throw at me, and to stay combative even while taking the measure of my inevitable decline. I repeat, this is no more than what a healthy person has to do in slower motion."

And finally, maybe the wisest of all the Other Voices: "A healthy attitude is contagious, but don't wait to catch it from others. Be a carrier." (Tom Stoppard, British playwright)

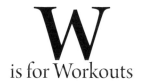

W

is for Workouts

I don't like to brag or toot my own horn or any of those other clichés that slyly refer to something you really do want to draw attention to, but my record concerning athletics is absolutely unsurpassed! When we played dodge ball in grammar school, I learned to head out early and run fast in order to avoid being hit. In high school I really surpassed my own abilities. In field hockey, I hugged the sidelines in order to avoid that darned puck. Basketball found me sort of loping along at the back of the pack in order to avoid having the ball actually passed to me, which would have required my having to dribble it. Volleyball wasn't bad as long as I managed to get on the right team so that I could spend most of my time standing still and serving the ball. I had a boyfriend in high school who was a tennis player, so I got hooked into spending a couple of sets on the tennis court until I managed to bend over to pick up a ball and hurt my back. Never could play tennis after that. Later I water skied once, and thereafter was in charge of the "skier down flag"—everyone in the boat has to earn their way, you see—and I moved up to snow skiing once at our cabin in the mountains. So you can plainly see that athletics have played a major role in my life.

When I got cancer, and ever since then, my many doctors and I have discussed the wide variety of workouts available to me, including the tremendous benefits these activities would provide me, especially as a long term survivor. The first thing they suggested was walking 30 minutes a day, three times a week. Unfortunately, that didn't work for me because I only like to walk in the forest where it's quiet and the dogs can run free. In fact, now that I mention it, that's another good reason why that 30 minute walking thing didn't work for me: it made my dogs nervous.

For a while I walked for 30 minutes on a treadmill I invested in, and that wasn't too terribly bad because while I walked I watched 30 minute long continuing education lectures, which met my requirement for continuing ed and resulted in my getting paid for walking. But then I got on some committees at the College and that counted as my continuing ed time, and there was no point in doing the treadmill thing anymore, so I gave it to my grandson.

For another little while I did a short 20 minute video thing every day, and that worked pretty well. That's when I lost enough weight to see that there was something wrong in my belly, and I tell you I'd still be doing that aerobic tape thing if only the second cancer hadn't interfered. Really. I would.

By the time I got through all the treatment and recovery for and from the second cancer, the 30 minute three day a week walk deal had changed to *10,000 steps per day!* Dr. Pirrucello explained how he managed to get in *10,000 steps every day* and how his pedometer worked and everything. I bought a pedometer, and I saw it in my car just the other day.

I always loved to dance, so I did try dancing during CNN commercials, but that involved an awful lot of getting up and sitting down and then getting up again, and pretty soon I was just too out of breath to dance.

About this time my sister and her husband joined a gym. My sister had injured her knee and had to have corrective surgery, and my brother-in-law had put on a few pounds he wanted to get rid of, so to the gym the pair of them a couple of days a week did go.

My sister and I talk every week. She is a psychotherapist and therefore very well aware of the nature of the human psyche. I'm confident that in the therapeutic process with her clients she is a gentle leader who sees her role as a facilitator to assist them in their journey of self-discovery. With me, she just tells me what I have to do. So, when the gym thing began to make her knee feel better and her husband began to shrink, the propaganda concerning the benefits of a gym workout began to come across not only the telephone lines but in internet e-mails as well. But I fought a good fight.

She said a workout at a gym would help me stay limber, and I told her I was plenty limber and could put my hands flat on the floor without bending my knees, even first thing in the morning.

She then said working out at the gym would increase my capacity for oxygen. I countered with the fact that we had done a baseline respiratory test, and my lung capacity was better than the doctor's.

She wouldn't be stopped, though. Next came the argument that working out at a gym would be a good cardio plan and would keep my heart healthy. I reminded her we'd put me through a major stress test, and my heart was in exceptional shape.

So far, you'll notice, I haven't been to the gym. I even mollified her a bit by looking into the senior fitness program at our local Y and giving her all the information. I even promised that after the first of the year (but I didn't say which year), I'd go to the new facility at the Y and check it out. Oh, I was proud of myself—just getting away with it was cool!

My sister and her husband went to visit their kids in Oregon over Christmas, and then I joined them at their home on New Year's so we could have our Christmas then. I opened the Native American story, and I loved it when I read it. I opened my "big" present—a really nice, soft sweater, perfect for the classroom. And then there was one more. Whatever could that be, I wondered. Well, you know very well it was a check for a Y membership, the first three months of the senior program and a trainer to develop my personal program. SNEAKY!!

But by that time I had done a great deal of research for this book, because I wanted to know what was happening to me. My ability to remember names was becoming much worse. I was losing my ability to recover my place in a lecture if a student interrupted me with an "off the wall" comment (which they do a lot). I found myself asking friends and family if I had already told or asked them something. I had trouble remembering not just dates, but even the day of the week.

I was having these awful physical problems involving a loss of energy to the point where I couldn't get out of bed. These times were accompanied by nausea and terrible, soaking sweats. I was becoming completely unable to tolerate heat, and would be dripping, as one of my students said, like a snow cone in Arizona, as I presented material in classes.

I was having trouble keeping my balance, and I found that when I went to meetings I had to focus so intently on what people were saying in order to understand them that I would be exhausted at the end and have to "take to my bed". And, I can say quite honestly, that I am not a person who "takes to her bed" without a darned good reason. (Even now, my mother wouldn't stand for it!)

Of course, my doctors and I were all trying to figure out what was going on, but everything we tested turned out better than normal, and we had just run out of ideas. I began to suspect that all of these complaints had something to do with my cancer treatment—although there were times that I was sure I was suffering a recurrence. Sure enough, by the time my sister gave me the gift to the gym, we were convinced that I was one of the many whose blood-brain barrier had been breached by chemotherapy, and that my brain had been injured.

This time I could not brush my sister off with a casual, "Oh my brain is just fine" because (1) it obviously isn't, (2) it's problematic enough that I've been researching possibilities for nearly two years, and (3) the problem is extensive enough among long term cancer survivors that I'm writing a book about it. Besides, I complained to her constantly about my memory problems and my fatigue. Oops!

When I got home after the holiday, I began to search my house frantically to find my hummingbird wings, and as soon as I did, those little guys got to churning again, and off we went to the new gym facilities that our Community Center leases to the YMCA. Now I go to senior fitness for strength training and balance work three times a week, and I go whenever I can to do the overall workout that the fitness trainer planned for me.

While fitting exercise into my routine, I'm keeping another Norman Cousins remark in mind to keep me going. He said, "Your heaviest artillery will be your will to live. Keep that big gun going!" And I figure if I could keep it going through two cancers and the treatment that went with them, I know absolutely I can keep it going to the gym, because despite all the "absent minded professor" jokes you may have heard, there's nothing at all funny about a professor who can't remember her subject, even with her lecture notes in her hands and even though she's been teaching it for more than 20 years!

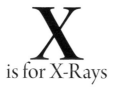

X

is for X-Rays

I can't remember when they handed out our dog tags at school, but I still have mine. They looked just like the dog tags soldiers wore, and they had our name, address, telephone number and blood type (!) on them. I don't remember that they told us anything about the danger of radiation in an atomic bomb attack, but they sure made us aware of a very dangerous thing called "the atomic bomb".

We had drills at school that were designed to save us from the bomb, but they only involved our getting under our desks in a yoga "child's pose", and resting our eyes on one arm while holding the other hand against the back of our necks. Then once a month the town atomic bomb warning sirens would go off, and people were supposed to run to the nearest "safe" spot, but since they always were tested at noon on the first Saturday of the month, it wasn't long before everyone was saying, "Oh, it's just the test" and going about their business.

There was lots of talk about the possibility of building (or digging) bomb shelters in back yards, and we had a big back yard, so my folks talked about it a good deal, trying to figure out how to make it big enough for all of us and our four neighbors. But nothing ever came of that.

I'm not sure what we were supposed to be afraid of as children, but we were definitely afraid. It could have been the explosion, the falling buildings, the mushroom cloud, or the fire, but it certainly wasn't radiation. We kids didn't have any idea what radiation was. We used to get our feet irradiated in these clever machines they had in shoe stores, and we loved looking at the bones in our tootsies. All we and our parents knew was that the machine would see to it that we got shoes that really fit.

My arm was x-rayed a lot when I broke it, and nobody said anything about that being a problem. You'll remember all the time I spent in the dentist's office, and every one of those trips involved x-rays. We had chest x-rays to make sure we didn't have tuberculosis, and I have faint memories of other medical procedures that involved x-rays. Everybody stayed in the room, so there was no hint of problems because the medical worker went into another room or stood behind a screen. I had no idea that these x-ray things had anything to do with radiation, and if I had, it wouldn't have made any difference, because I didn't have a clue as to what radiation was.

So, I'm not sure when I became aware that radiation was dangerous to my health. It must have gradually worked its way into my consciousness as I grew older. I do remember being very shocked when it was announced that the shoe store x-ray machines were bad. And I've read in the last few years about folks being unaware of the amount of radiation people could be exposed to before it became hazardous and, as a result, probably zapping people much more than was necessary to get a clear picture.

Somewhere along the line, though, I got very clear on the fact that if you got cancer, you probably would have to have something called radiation (no connection made to x-rays), and that if you had to have this radiation, it would be very, very bad.

So by the time cancer became part of my life, I had an idea of what radiation was, how it worked, and why cancer patients had to have it. At least I wasn't totally in the dark!

During my first visit to Radiology at the Med Center, I asked the technician why radiation would make patients feel exhausted, which was the only warning I had received about it. He said they didn't know, but they figured there was a psychological component. So I decided I would treat it like a job. I would get up every morning, drive into town, have my treatment and come home. I had just six weeks off between semesters, so I didn't have to worry about teaching, and I think if I had, that fatigue problem would have shown itself. But as it worked out, all I HAD to do during those six weeks was have my radiation treatment. And I did just fine.

I did just fine, that is, except for the huge radiation burn I got from my treatments! I'm happy to report that it didn't make me tired, but oh, my, how it did hurt. It was so big and raw that it hurt to look at it! The radiation oncologist prescribed an ointment, which didn't seem to help it much, but she didn't mention that I probably shouldn't be wearing my bra over the burn in the hot summer that is our climate. So, by the time I had an appointment with Dr. Pirruccello, who said, "You can't cover that with clothes!" my summer class had started, and I was in pain. But still, I argued that I couldn't go to work without my prosthesis, and Dr. P argued just as strongly that I didn't have a choice! So for the next six weeks I taught self-consciously hunched over my lectern, and imagined that my students were wondering why I didn't walk around the room as I usually do. But the burn healed, and the class went well, so it all turned out in the end.

My final lesson in radiation came only two or three years ago. I had my regular appointment with Dr. Alali and asked him if we were going to do a CT scan, and he said, "Oh, no, Patricia. You've already had more than enough radiation." Another oops! Somewhere along the line during all of this cancer stuff, I had missed the message that the really, really bad thing about radiation is that it can give you cancer as well as treat it, and if you get way too much radiation, it can kill you.

Well, then. My radiation education was complete. So, if you had radiation with your cancer treatment, be sure you tell any new doctors about it, so that they use some other process that doesn't involve radioactive material if they possibly can.

Y
is for Yours Alone

Cancer is not a competition. Your cancer is yours and yours alone. No one else has the same kind of cancer, type of cancer, size of tumor in the same place at the same age in the same socio-economic status as you. No one can "share" your pain. Bill Clinton is probably the only person in the world who could get away with saying, "I feel your pain", but he was talking about money!

The late, but never to be forgotten, Humphrey Bogart of "Casa Blanca" movie fame was married to Lauren Bacall. Theirs was a great affair of the heart, and they were together until lung cancer took him from her. Here's what Ms. Bacall says about illness: "A man's illness is his private territory and, no matter how much he loves you and how close you are, you stay an outsider. You are healthy".

How many times have you heard, "Oh, I know what you mean …." when you've mentioned something about your illness, your treatment, or your long term after effects? My guess, based on my own experience is that you've heard that almost as often as you've heard, "GET OVER IT!" The first just sounds more kindly and compassionate than the second.

The loneliness of cancer is evidenced by the number of support groups, especially online support groups, that are available to cancer survivors, particularly those who have been through breast cancer. When no one else seems to understand, we can turn to the privacy and anonymity (if we choose) of our computers.

Our pain is measured by the little smiling to frowning faces with their accompanying numbers that show on the chart hanging on the exam room's wall. But my smiling face might well be your frowning face, and who are we to question the other?

Why even talk about the size of our tumors, the nature of our surgery, how we responded to chemo or how radiation affected us? We're all different, and our disease, though carrying the same name, is different. Our responses to both the disease itself and the situation in which we find ourselves are not like the responses of anyone else. Recognizing that we are similar, only similar, is, I think, a matter of respect.

I referred before to Lao Tzu and the *Tao de Ching*. Let's look at that fine little book once again:

> Simplicity, patience, compassion.
> These three are your greatest treasures.
> Simple in actions and thoughts, you return to the source of being.
> Patient with both friends and enemies, you accord with the way things are.
> Compassionate toward yourself, you reconcile all beings in the world.

And perhaps even more importantly, let us become beautiful people and help others become beautiful people as they are described by the late Elizabeth Kubler-Ross whose great work on death and dying is the foundation for our understanding of illness that has the potential to be terminal. She said, "The most beautiful people we have known are those who have known defeat, known suffering, known struggle, known loss, and have found their way out of the depths. These persons have an appreciation, a sensitivity, and an understanding of life that fills them with compassion, gentleness, and a deep loving concern. Beautiful people do not just happen."

Let us become what we would like others to be and in the process help change cancer centers, infusion labs, and radiation departments all over the world into better places. Let us remember that we all are suffering and struggling, and that's enough to know. Beyond that, let us bring nothing to bear on the discussion but compassion so that we can become simple, beautiful people.

Z

is for Zephyr's Transformation

The story of the west wind is a story of transformation, which I think is really appropriate for cancer patients. In Greek mythology, the god of the west wind is called Zephyrus. He was the companion of Boreas, god of the north wind. The two were "savage and baleful, and took great pleasure in brewing storms and tossing the waves of the sea". They were said to live in the mountainous regions of Thrace, north of Greece, and they caused nothing but trouble. The great English poet, Shelley, in his "Ode to the West Wind" calls to Zephyrus, saying "Destroyer and preserver; hear, oh hear!", thus recording in more modern times the dual nature of Zephyrus.

Ovid tells us a story about the two aspects of Zephyrus in his *Fasti,* where the nymph, Chloris, speaks : " It was spring, I wandered; Zephyrus [the West Wind] saw me, I left. He pursues, I run : he was the stronger; and Boreas [the North Wind] gave his brother full rights of rape.. But he [Zephyrus] makes good the rape by naming me his bride, and I have no complaints about my marriage. I enjoy perpetual spring: the year always shines, trees are leafing, the soil always fodders. I have a fruitful garden in my dowered fields, fanned by breezes, fed by limpid fountains. My husband filled it with well-bred flowers, saying: `Have jurisdiction of the flower, goddess.'"

Perhaps it was this marriage to Chloris, gracious nymph of Spring, or maybe the birth of their child, Carpus, whose name means fruit, that caused Zephyrus' violent disposition to soften. We don't know for certain. But from an angry, destructive god, he became a sweet-scented wind that blew gently across the fields of Elysium. And in honor of this transformed Zephyrus, the Athenians consecrated an altar to him at Eleusis.

Now, to my way of thinking, there's no better story to serve as a metaphor for cancer and its treatment than that of Zephyrus. Indeed, Zephyrus is described as "baleful", and a synonym for that word is malignant! Like Zephyrus, the savage cancer seeks to cause great storms in our lives and threatens to destroy us. The aggressive surgery, chemotherapy and radiation steal our lives and keep us in dark, solitary caves for a year before we begin to see a softening and feel the hope represented in the newly transformed, gentle Zephyr.

Apuleius, in *The Golden Ass*, tells us a story of the new god and his ways: "But as Psyche wept in fear and trembling on that rocky eminence [where she had been left as a sacrifice to what she believed was a monster], Zephyrus' kindly breeze with its soft stirring wafted the hem of her dress to and fro, and with tranquil breath bore her slowly downward [from the mountain-side]. She glided down in the bosom of the flower-decked turf in the valley below [and the hidden palace of Eros]."

And, like Zephyrus, we are transformed. We are the same people we were before cancer, and we are completely different. We possess a dual nature—survivor and patient. It would be wonderful if we could live now in eternal Spring, but we must deal with the long term effects of our treatment. They are not comfortable. The paths they might take are unknown, and the ultimate outcomes are a mystery. We don't even know who among us will sustain them or to what extent.

Even so, we have to honor our struggles by thinking always of the transformational qualities of the gentle west wind of ancient myth. We must vow not to let the old, powerful Zephyrus consume us again. Rather, we must think of the sweet smelling, kindly Zephyr who rescued Psyche (Self) and carried her gently to the flower filled meadow. That's the image that will guide us through. If we hold on to Zephyr's tranquil breath, we will survive the long term after effects, too. We will be in that place the ancient Roman stoic, Seneca, describes—that place "Where meadows lie which Zephyrus soothes with his dew-laden breath and calls forth the herbage of the spring."

And when we lose our connection to that meadow, we can recall the words of John Masefield, former Poet Laureate of Great Britain, in his poem "The West Wind", where in the second stanza he gives voice to Zephyrus, saying:

Larks are singing in the west, brother, above the green wheat,
So will ye not come home, brother, and rest your tired feet?
I've a balm for bruised hearts, brother, sleep for aching eyes,
Says the warm wind, the west wind, full of birds' cries.

References

Bangley, Bernard, Ed., Nearer to the Heart of God: Daily Readings with the Christian Mystics, Paraclete Press, Brewster: 2005, ISBN 1-55725-417-6

Campbell, Joseph, Ed., *The Portable Jung*, Viking Press, New York: 1971 ISBN 670-01070-7

Crespi, Catherine M., Ganz, Patricia A., Petersen, Laura, Castillo, Adrienne and Caan, Bette, "Refinement and Psychometric Evaluation of the Impact of Cancer Scale", JNCI, Vol 100, Issue 21, November 5, 2008, http://jnci.oxfordjournals.org

Emerson, David, Hopper, Elizabeth, PhD, *Overcoming Trauma Through Yoga*, North Atlantic Books, Berkeley and The Trauma Center at Justice Resource Institute, Inc., Boston: 2010, ISBN 978-1-55643-969-8

Fields, R. Douglas, "White Matter Matters", Scientific American, March, 2008, pp 54-61

Gotay, Carolyn C. and Pagano, Ian S., "Assessment of Survivor Concerns (ASC): A Newly Proposed Brief Questionnaire", Health and Quality of Life Outcomes, 2007; 5:15, http://www.hqlo.com/content/5/1/15

Fincher, Susanne F., *Creating Mandalas*, Shambhala, Boston & London: 1991 ISBN 0-87773-646-4

Fontana, David, *Meditating with Mandalas*, Duncan Baird Publishers, London: 2005 ISBN 13-9-781844-831401

Foster, Richard J, Grffin, Emilie, Eds., *Spiritual Classics: Selected Readings on the Twelve Spiritual Disciplines*, Harper One, New York: 2000, ISBN 978-0-06-062872-7

Graves, Robert (Introduction), *New Larousse Encyclopedia of Mythology*, Hamlyn, London: 1968, ISBN 0-600-02420-2

Hirsch, E. D., Jr., Kett, Joseph F. and Trefil, James, Eds., *The Dictionary of Cultural Literacy: What Every American Needs to Know*, 2d Ed., Houghton Mifflin, New York: 1993 ISBN 0-395-65597-8

Huxley, Aldous, *The Perennial Philosophy: An Interpretation of the Great Mystics, East and West,* Perennial Classics Edition, published by Perennial, an imprint of HarperCollins Publishers, New York: 2004 ISBN 0-06-057058-X

Inman, Mason, "White Matter Listens In", Scientific American Mind, Aug/Sep 2007. Vol.18, Issue 4, p8, http://web.ebscohost.com/chost/delivery?sid

Johnson, Glen, Traumatic Brain Injury Survival Guide, Version 1.2,e-book, www.tbiguide.com

Lao Tzu, *The Tao Te Ching*. Dale, Ralph Alan Trans., Sacred Wisdom Series, Watkins Publishing, London: 2007 ISBN 978-1-84293-123-3

Luke, Helen M., *Woman, Earth and Spirit: The Feminine in Symbol and Myth*, Crossroad Publishing, New York: 1990, ISBN0-8245-0633-2

MacReady, Norra, "Chemotherapy Can Affect Cognitive Function (Neurology)", Internal Medicine News, March 1, 2005, Vol 38, Iss 5, p 38

Mayo Clinic Staff, "When Cancer Returns: How to Cope with Cancer Recurrence, Mayo Foundation for Medical Education and Research (MFMER), Rochester: 2011 "Cancer Survivors: Reconnecting with Loved Ones After Treatment", MFMER, Rochester: 2011

Merton, Thomas, *The Collected Poems of Thomas Merton*, New Directions Publishing, New York: 1977, ISBN 0-8112-0769-2

Merton, Thomas, Shannon, William H. Ed., *The Inner Experience: Notes on Contemplation*, Harper, San Francisco, 2003 ISBN 0-06-053928-3

Metzger, Bruce M., Coogan, Michael D. Eds., *The Oxford Companion to the Bible*, Oxford University Press, New York: 1993, ISBN 0-19-50-504645-5

Morris, Mary, Grant, Marcia, Lynch, James, "Patient-reported Family Distress Among Long-term Cancer Survivors", Cancer Nursing, Vol. 30, No. 1, 2007

National Cancer Institute, National Institutes of Health, <u>Facing Forward:
Life After Cancer Treatment</u>, "Body Changes and Intimacy",
www.nationalcancerinstitute.com

National Cancer Institute, National Institutes of Health, <u>Facing Forward:
Life After Cancer Treatment</u>, "Social and Work Relationships", www.
nationalcancerinstitute.com

Phillips, Dorothy Berkley, Howes, Elizabeth Boyden and Nixon, Lucille, *The
Choice is Always Ours*, A Re-Quest Book, published by Pyramid Publications for The Theosophical Publishing House, Wheaton: 1975

Piercy, Marge, *What Are Big Girls Made Of?*, Alfred A. Knopf, New York:
2007 ISBN 0-679-76594-8 *Available Light*, Alfred A. Knopf, New York:
1988, ISBN 0-394-75691-6 *The Moon is Always Female*, Alfred A. Knopf,
New York: 2008. ISBN 0-394-73859-4 *Stone, Paper, Knife*, Alfred A.
Knopf, New York, 1983, ISBN 0-394-71219-6 *The Twelve-Spoked Wheel
Flashing*, Alfred A. Knopf, New York: 1978, ISBN 0-394-73488-2 Editor,
Early Ripening: American Women's Poetry Now, Pandora, New York: 1987
ISBN 0-86358-141-2

PubMed Health, National Institutes of Health, "MS: Demyelinating
Disease", A.D.A.M. Medical Encyclopedia, Atlanta: 2011, last reviewed
8/5/2010

Raffa, Robert B. and Tallarida, Ronald J. Eds, *Chemo Fog: Cancer Chemotherapy-Related Cognitive Impairment*. Springer Science+Business Media,
LLC, New York: 2010 ISBN 978-1-4419-6305-5

Revised Standard Version, 2d Ed., *Holy Bible:* 1972, Thomas Nelson, Inc.,
Nashville

Silverman, Dan, M.D., PhD, and Idelle Davidson, *Your Brain After Chemo:
A Practical Guide to Lifting the Fog and Getting Back Your Focus*, Da Capo
Press, Cambridge: 2009 ISBN 978-0-73821391-0

Susuki, Kelichiro, MD, PhD, et al, "Myelin: A Specialized Membrane for Cell
Communication", <u>Nature Education 3(9):</u>59, www.nature.com/scitable/
topicpage/myelin

Van den Beuken-van Everdingen, Marieke H. J., et al, "Concerns of Former
Breast Cancer Patients About Disease Recurrence: A Validation and
Prevalence Study", <u>Psycho-Oncology</u>, 2008, Wiley InterScience
(www.interscience.wiley.com)

Walker, Barbara G., *The Woman's Dictionary of Symbols & Sacred Objects*, Harper, San Francisco, 1988, ISBN: 0-06-250923-1

Walker, Barbara G., *The Woman's Encyclopedia of Myths and Secrets*, Harper & Row: San Francisco: 1983, ISBN 0-06-250925-X

Leading: Norman Cousins, http://www harvardsquarelibrary.org/unitarians/cousins.html

Spirituality: Ernest Holms, http://ernestholmes.wwwhubs.com/

Useful: http://www.cancer.med.umich.edu/living/quotes.shtml

Voices: http://www.cancer.med.umich.edu/living/quotes.shtml

Zephyr: http://www.theoi.com/Titan/AnemosZephyros.html
http://famouspoetsandpoems.com/poets/john_masefield/poems/15257
http://rpo.library.utoronto.ca/poem/1902.html

Made in the USA
San Bernardino, CA
09 December 2013